What My Brain Has Taught Me

A teaching memoir of hopeful service
for those living with and through brain tumors, surgery and/or injuries
as well as for those who love and care for them.

Rev. Regina Maria Cross, MS

Published by Curly Girl Publications, Tahlequah, Oklahoma
curlygirlpublications.com

reginamaria@curlygirlpublications.com

Copyright 2020 by Curly Girl Publications

First Edition

A portion of the proceeds of the sale of this book will be donated to the
American Brain Tumor Association (ABTA)

ISBN: 978-1-09834-280-7 (print)
ISBN: 978-1-09834-281-4 (eBook)

Manufactured in The United States of America
Cover Design
God, Regina Maria & Ken Cross and Levina Patterson
Artwork
Ken Cross

In The Beginning

DEDICATION

To God, Thank You for saying; "Yes, Live".
To Jesus and Elizabeth who have never left me alone.

To my Beloved Kenny who lives truth daily
and has never left my side nor right brain.

To Drs. Arthur Kobrine, M.D. and Ladislau Steiner, MD, PhD,
Neurosurgeons par excellence.
I am here because they were there for me.

To Patricia Beamer O'Sullivan, my Brain Buddy Bookend, my "Beamer",
who knew if we put our heads together, we could save the world.
"If they'd only listen."

To all who are mentioned between the pages.

To all who are presently living with, to those who have survived,
and to those who will experience brain trauma in their life
as my intention has been in writing this book
to be of service to you and your caregivers needs.

Remember:
"You're braver than you believe,
stronger than you seem, and smarter than you think."

Christopher Robin

ACKNOWLEDGMENT

To Spirit who inspired the laying of language in the most magnificent way of words.

To my beloved husband and best friend, Kenny, who has lovingly endured the journey and now has artfully created each illustration breathing life into the stick people in my head.

To Shawn Sizer who got the book ball rolling. This book exists because of his encouraging words after hearing my end of a deeply heartfelt phone conversation.

To my soul sista', Mary Ann Owens, whose brilliant brain saw the birthing of the Card Deck.

To Jennifer Palmer, who without her tears, my stories would not have been told.

To Robert Schulte, PC, whose loving legalese covered my ass. Hehehehehe....

To the Tahlequah Oklahoma Writers group who listened, critiqued, guided and held my hand leading me through the "Business of Booking" as those who have gone before.

To all my Editors:

My cousin Rosemary Rest whose detail is to die for but then, "She'd have to kill me." My cousin Cecilia Forbes who gave me the idea of flipping chapters. My pro, Kris Cooper, who did a fabulous job while keeping my voice and teaching me "The word big means big." My aha moment regarding capitalization.

To writers I have forever loved and to those I recently have met through conferences and workshops. Their foot placement before me allowed an easier trek up the mountain toward publication. Thank you, Nikki Hanna, my "saging sista" wordsmith.

To all those helpful through the reading of the manuscript prior to publication as it is their insightful assessment, suggestions and reviews that helped catapult the book into existence.

To my Angel Agent, manager and promoter, Randy Gibson of RDG Communications who makes magic as if it is the ordinary of life. Big love and hugs to Charity Rene Strawn for bringing us together.

Know I am eternally grateful for all of you and the assistance you so willingly gave through your hearts and souls being a part of this plan of service to humanity.

You are ALL Awesome! (Capital "A" plus exclamation point)

TABLE OF CONTENTS

Chapter Three: After Brain Surgery (ABS)
Me and My Brain Living The Good Life Most of the Time 79

Chapter Four: Again With The Brain Tumor 111

FOREWORD

What My Brain Has Taught Me by Rev. Regina Maria Cross, MS is a beautifully written story of courage, transformation, and healing. A brain tumor diagnosis of right temporal lobe meningioma was devastating for Regina Maria. Such a diagnosis required deep courage, strength, and faith. Through her profoundly inspiring and touching story, she shares the wisdom she gained on her path to living a life that nurtures body, mind, and the spirit, and awakens one to the joy of living. Throughout her book, she provides helpful words of love and encouragement, and describes how to live life more meaningfully and fully. As a retired hospice chaplain, I would highly recommend this book to anyone who is dealing with life threatening brain cancer.

Rev. Katherine James Klemstine, D.Min.

INTRODUCTION

Dear Reader,

Thank you for picking up my book. Thank you even bigger if you have bought it. Thank you to those who have given it as a gift. It is in the realm of gifting I hope it is identified. This book is nothing magical, nothing medical yet my hope is, it is mindful in Service. It is my gift to you for surviving a very scary chapter in your span of days, for your courageous one step at a time moving forward living life again from a higher point of view. It is my gift to those who love and care for you during the journey navigating through the unknown. My hope is by virtue of the contents of its pages you will find inspiration, new thought, a smile, a prayer, an encouraging way of accepting your new normal as you re-create your authentic self.

Stories are sprinkled through the lessons within *What My Brain Has Taught Me* because I met a woman one day who made me realize many of our stories are the same.

When we hear our story coming from another there is the realization that we are all connected by a fine web of adventures meaning we are not alone through a dark night of the soul journey. There is Heavenly help and Earthly assistance as we grope through the navigation of whence, we know not. Inside Part One *Once Upon My Time Stories* there are narratives, I know you will recognize as your own, different names, dates and times yet you have lived them. Hopefully there in front of you as you read or are read to, know my intention is to honor your story as well.

Held within the contents of Part Two *My Brain Has Taught Me These Things* you will find tidbits of information helpful as you travel your road of recovery, guidance of care which took me years and some decades to acknowledge as such. Self-Attentiveness in the realms of: Your blessed head, your spirit, your attitude, your emotions, your movement, resources and so much more.

Please do have fun with the *Today I Count My I AM Blessings* Card Deck. Hopefully they will inspire you to believe just how great thou art through the awareness of Blessings coming your way on a daily basis.

The blank Personal Journal *Look What I Can Do* is all about you because you deserve it to be.

Now, it is time for my book to do its work right along with you.

My book is a teaching memoir of survival. My book of service is timeless. It is about staying fully alive in your body, your mind, your heart, and your soul, realizing the gift you have been given living with and through a brain tumor, surgery, or injury as you accept and appreciate the Blessing you are. It is brimming with soulful wisdom and heartfelt humor. It is chock-full of information your Neuro people may not have. I want you to be inspired through the journey, be excited about the Aha's as they may work for you, laugh through the concession of this is truly goofy, praise and feel gratitude for that which is real and smile big, for you are a living, breathing miracle right here, right now all by yourself.

Namaste,
Rev. Regina Maria Cross, MS

A NEW DAY DAWNING

A sacred time 6:00am, as all time is. My time of birth. The time of waking preparing me for a craniotomy. I am alive because God said "Yes Live." I am blessed to breathe into another day this side of life, rebirthing the bliss through ordinary living. Deeply caring for that which truly matters. Then I am alive as I am meant to be.

AN IRISH BLESSING

May you never forget what is worth remembering
Nor
Ever remember what is best forgotten
Amen

PART ONE

Once Upon My Time Stories

Chapter One

Before Brain Surgery (BBS)
My Brain This Side of Life
Or
It's All In Your Head

Starts with a "B" * October 19, 1989

Kenny and I woke with excitement in our hearts as this was the day, October 19, 1989, that finally, after six years of diagnostic testing and surgeries, we just may have answers to our baby making journey. So, we felt assured he need not be with me for the last of testing that day. As his sister, Jeanne, was visiting from Florida and she and I were close, she traveled with me to the hospital for what we thought would be an effortless day with reason to celebrate by days end. Following a check-it-off-the-list testing procedure called HSG—Major Ouch!— she assisted me down the hallway to the MRI capsule like a Girl Scout helping an old lady cross the street.

Why an MRI? It was a fact, my prolactin level (a hormone released from the anterior pituitary gland that stimulates milk production after childbirth) was high enough I could be the official neighborhood wet nurse. Our beloved Endocrinologist Reproductive Specialist, Dr. Christos Mastroyannis, felt an MRI was in order checking for the possibility of a pituitary tumor, which, as he stated, is a relatively simple fix. All right let's go for it and get on with making mine and Kenny's babies.

So, relieved to be lying down after my morning procedure, I was slipped into the capsule. I sighed a big sigh, thinking; *I'm clueless as to what is happening, but it can't be any weirder than what I have already been through. And this is it! We will have all our answers very soon.* The alien noise began, and it was all I could do not to laugh out loud as visions of National Geographic Hooters Women danced in my head to the rhythm of the magnetic drumming. After what seemed a very long time the tech came bustling in grabbing my right arm as the capsule bed slid out toward him and with a syringe the size of Manhattan said, "You've got something in there. Something in your head." He shot me with some orange goo and hurled the rolling table into reverse throwing me back into what seemed like something akin to a NASA Space Capsule now ready for blast off. My thought regarding his electrified comment; "You've got something in there." *OK, one would hope. Of course, I have something in there. It's called a brain!* My choices here are to panic or relax into the idea that I have more time all to myself for meditation. I chose the latter.

When he pulled me out, I became wrapped in the entire night's bizarre episode of "Excuse me? Say what? This can't be true!" Before my jelly-like legs had rounded the table's edge, before my near numb feet touched the floor, this crazy man was saying; "You have a brain tumor and we've got to get it out right now." Well, that just did not register even in the slightest. *This guys a nut.* Then I saw my sister-in-law's face and became puzzled and frightened inside.

He rushed me out of the MRI room so fast, I barely had time to snatch her hand to come with me keeping me safe from this quack. He was just a little too stimulated and the situation a little too surreal for me as he took my hand bolting me into the reception area of the X-ray Department waiting room full of weary people. Sitting me down, throwing a woman's magazine (I figured that because there was a woman baking cookies on the front cover) into my lap repeating over and over "Read something to me." "Excuse me?" "Read! Read something now!"

This guy is totally freaking me out. I had come to the hospital that day for the last of the "baby questing" testing procedures thrilled by the idea that now Kenny and I would have our answers leading to our next step toward the direction of our baby in arms. Meanwhile this near hysterical man is telling me crazy things and demanding I read. Fear jolted through me unknown to anyone other than Kenny at the time. My inner guts just wanted to scream at him, *I can't read!* Instead, I had to quickly be clever once again in life hiding shame while my outer demeanor was trying desperately to hold onto some semblance of reality. Looking up into his anxious eyes, doing my best to appear calm while closing the magazine, I quietly stated, "I'm sorry, you just told me I have a brain tumor (at which time everyone in the room turned and stared). I have no interest in reading to you."

He hurriedly grabbed my wrist, again, as I tried to grab the phone off the receptionist desk saying, "I need to call my husband." "There's no time for that now. We have to get you into surgery." I grabbed Jeanne's hand, as he pushed his way past those waiting in line at the reception desk and into the Light Room where only doctors, nurses and doctors' kids are allowed. Ahhh, now I get it. This guy thinks he has found something on my MRI. Not only did he actually see something on an MRI, which must be just a little exciting for him, but he found it in Dr. Alfred John Suraci's, the Chief of Surgeons daughter's head. He wants me to know he knows everything he has ever learned in school so I can tell Dad and he can show Dad how brilliant he is. Holy MRI! Why else would we be going deep into the secret inner sanctum where he throws a galaxy of semi-translucent images unlike anything I'd seen before up on the Light Boards. He said, "See! You have a brain tumor, and we need to get it out right now." *Oh, yea, I know what you're looking at. Sure, I see it clearly now, of course. Everybody step back from the nut case. This is absolutely no way to treat a patient! Someone get him away from me! Someone save me!"*

While in my frigid (which is no reference to our baby questing by the way), I still have not exhaled since you first seized my life stance, doctor faces that I knew well from visits in my parents' home suddenly started appearing over the tops of their seclusion isolation cubicles. They too began to hold their breath. *Oh, this is so not working for me.... easy day supposed to be an easy day.*

Suddenly, and quite literally, I felt a Brilliance of Light Rays, much like the Chaplet of Divine Mercy painting, shine behind me, embracing every fiber of my Being. I turned to witness Dr. Christos busting through the door with a fused look of sheer anger on his face toward the tech while complete savior toward me. Christos took my hand and along with Jeanne stole me away from cuckoo, loopy, fruitcake man, into the cloaked back halls that only hospital personnel and some of their children knew existed. We walked in silence through the long beige tunnel into the elevator to the third floor. *Third Floor: lingerie, ladies' purses, endocrinologist fertility specialist's office, and talk of a brain tumor. Please exit safely.* Again, heading down the halls of precisely, indescribable beige, his fingers entwined in mine were the only thing keeping me grounded. And yet, I could feel his terror of truth.

This dear, sweet man needs a laugh. I know I do. I looked at him with a smile on my face and said, "OK, came in for a baby, I'm hearing brain tumor. Starts with a B, so possibly someone got things mixed up? And speaking of mixed up maybe they aren't my MRI's. Maybe they are someone else's. Not that I want them to be someone else's but maybe..." While watching his face, I could tell he was trying ever so hard to spring up a smile, but it wasn't working.

Hours passed in the office with Christos, Dr. Robert Simmons, the Medical Director of Providence Hospital in Washington, D.C. and Jeanne as I was trying my best to grasp what was being said. How am I to go home with this news and tell my Beloved, "Nope, no baby, but, I do have a brain tumor." What about my parents? I know I'm thirty-nine but no matter how old I get, I will always be one of their babies. If we do not tell them tonight, when Dad walks into Providence Hospital tomorrow morning for his rounds everyone but he will know. Also true for my baby brother, Michael and baby sister, Pattie, both of whom are nurses here. This truly is bizarro-world.

For five... count them five... years Kenny and I had gone to doctor after doctor after doctor trying to find reasoning for my horrific intense headaches. As the day grew longer it was as if my head were in a vice that just kept tightening with every passing hour. One doctor actually thought I was making it up, no big deal, take a few aspirin, or actually if it will make you feel better, he did not mean physically, I will give you a prescription for Naprosyn. Then he patted me on the head. Really, did you not hear me? Painful! I'm having seizures! Once on the way to another baby questing doctor appointment before we met Christos, I started to seizure in the car. After arriving for my appointment, I told the doctor reminding him sarcastically as if it would make a difference that he had to legally tell me I could not drive anymore. His response while he continued looking down at his clipboard was, "Don't drive anymore." He continued, "Now let's..." "Seriously, do I pay you for that? I need help." We needed help and no one helped. For five years, no one helped. They all pretended I was not in my right mind. Come to find out, on this day of expected elation, I had a right temporal lobe brain tumor nearly the size of a well-fed turbo golf ball now impinging parietal as well as the occipital lobes of my brain.

I will never forget the look on Kenny's face nor the embrace he held me in when I told him the news. Simultaneously, Jeanne was telling her husband, Ken's parents and other siblings. At the same time, Dr. Robert Simmons had already called my parents' home and spoken with my Mom. Thank God my baby sister, Pattie, was there beside her. Robert would call back after Dad's arrival home from his long hours of doctor day.

The last thing Dad said to me that night was, "Baby Girl, if we have to go out of state, if we have to leave the country, you will have the very best in the very best environment." In that moment I knew how Blessed Kenny and I were to have such a weight lifted from our shoulders as we stepped through Door Number 2 of unknown territory.

Within 24 hours my MRI's had traveled throughout the United States. Within 3 days they had journeyed around the world. Ninety-nine percent of all answers came right back here to Washington, DC highlighting a Dr. Arthur Kobrine, who as a young intern, saved James Brady's life the day he and President Reagan were shot. More Blessings. More story...

Three Mornings After The Long Nights Before

"I don't know where I'm going."

"When will you be back?"

"I haven't a clue. If I don't know where I'm going, I don't know when I'll be back."

I was driving Kenny crazy. He knows me well. I am not the type to just get up and go by any means. I can be as spontaneous as the next person as long as I know ahead of time. So, this walking into his barn-studio announcing that I am going for a drive three mornings after the last three long nights before, after being told I have a brain tumor the size of an overblown golf ball, was way out of my definition of impulsive.

"I'm coming with you"

"No you're not. I just need to go away."

"Go away? Are you coming back?"

"I don't know what I'm doing." Kenny had no choice but to pull up his big boy pants and watch me drive away.

Up until that day, since the moment after I told Kenny the news and his response was so brave, I was like a suction cup on him and his spirit. I was in a numb space outside myself.

I still haven't a clue as to where I went. I drove country roads at first known, then unknown for hours. Nine hours to be exact. I drove. I cried. I screamed. I stared holding my breath. I thought thoughts in literal, in imagination, in different scenarios of this and that, of what if's and what if nots. I cried some more. Stared some more. And now and again I could feel myself take a long deep breath from my solar plexus, up through my heart, my chest, my throat, through my face, and into my eyes. I talked to my inner self and sometimes just to myself, as to who should be in charge of what, my will, my funeral, and my vegetative self should that happen.

Who should take care of Kenny? Who will help him take care of Beau, our Bearded Collie, best puppy dog? He won't need anybody to help him take care of Beau. They are inside each other's skin even if they are different species. What if Kenny had not come back almost a year ago after his sabbatical? Would I have told him? Well, that was easy...And No. I have a real thing about anybody being in my life out of obligation.

For whatever reason I disappeared for the day, through exhaustion on every level of my being physical, emotional, mental and spiritual I was now ready to turn the car around, put it on auto pilot toward Belvoir Farms in Crownsville, Maryland, and ride on up the road to the barn where Kenny still had the lights burning and Beau waited on the floor by the door. I needed to fall into a heap of nothing as I had spent it all that day, and the only Being on earth I wanted to fall into was Kenny.

As I started up the mile dirt road, Jeanne, Kenny's sister, who had been with me all day on October 19 as a walking blessing, was taking an evening stroll. She waved. We met up. I stopped the car, put it in park and got out. She came toward me with her ever easy eyes and calm smile. Facing each other we took hands and, as we did, I broke down.

"Oh, My God, Jeanne! All my hair is going to be gone! Kenny and I decided on our Honeymoon I was going to grow it out to waist length. I'm almost there, and it's all going to be gone! And it's so stupid I'm even thinking about that cause I could lose my life, but Noooooo, I'm worried about losing my hair. That's crazy."

Jeanne quietly stroked my hair with both hands. Then her left hand caressed my right check. She gazed at me and in her soft voice said something I have never forgotten. Something I have integrated into my own intimate compassion both personally and professionally.

"Honey, that's not stupid. You cannot see your brain tumor when you look in the mirror. Your hair symbolizes your brain tumor." It was one of those moments that all else stops as Grace allows you to take in all that has just been given to you. Jeanne took the keys from me and drove us the rest of the way up to Ken's barn-studio. As we got out, she turned and walked on toward Mother and Grampie's home as I entered Kenny's art world. When he turned to see who was coming in the wide wooden door, the look across his face was complete relief and a little bit of boy across the room at the high school dance.

His hug was a rush. The perfect rush I needed.

"You OK?"

"I am right now."

"Where did you go?"

"I haven't a clue...And everywhere."

And so it was, three days after the long nights before, was my first ever: I'm just taking off unrehearsed for places unknown. There was nothing relaxed, free and easy, unselfconscious, uninhibited, impetuous, or unthinking about it. But it was natural, instinctive, exploratory, deeply intuitive and very much needed.

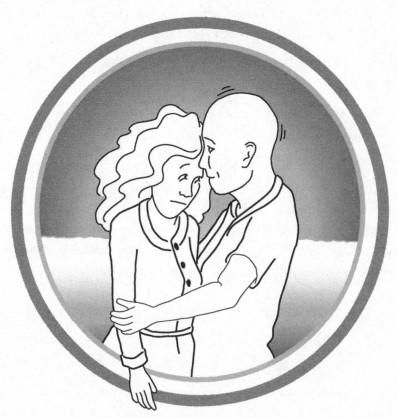

A First For Everything.

A First For Everything * November 7, 1989

Being November in Washington, D.C. I am almost certain it was a cold day but, in truth, I couldn't tell you for sure. I also have no memory of how we arrived at Dr. Arthur Kobrine's office. Did we, Kenny and I, drive by ourselves or did we drive with my Mom and Dad? We must have driven with my parents. Neither Ken nor I remember the drive back home. I do not remember the afternoon or evening after my first consult appointment.

What I do remember is almost everything else: What I was wearing, a very professional grown-up two-piece suit in beige linen with a fine feminine cut to it. The absolute fear that pulsed through every fiber of my being. From their facial expressions and their hands, it was obvious the same fear was pumping through Kenny, my Mom and my Dad. The walls were beige. There was a framed article hanging on the wall about Dr. Arthur Kobrine and how he saved James Brady the day he was shot alongside President Reagan. Dad stood and read it as we waited in the reception room. I pretended to do the same doing my very best imitation of being at ease. The office was quiet yet busy. A woman, bald as a baby's butt, kept watching me, me, with the waist length dark curly hair.

We were called into Dr. Arthur Kobrine's office. I do not remember much about what was discussed while my parents were in there. It is a near guarantee that the Q&A between Dad and Dr. Kobrine was high level doctor talk. My yellow pad with blue-green lines of 40 questions lay neatly upon the lap of my polished beige linen skirt waiting it's turn for inquiry. Prior to our leave that morning, I had told Kenny when the time came for me to ask questions about my survival, I was going to ask my parents to leave the room. I know they know things. Dad's a doctor; Mom's a nurse. They know things. And, I am their daughter. I will always be their daughter.

My parents, the people who bought me into this world, do not need to hear the question: Am I going to die? They do not need to know these things right now, in front of me hearing them. The time came. I stood and requested they leave, "There are just a few private things Kenny and I want to discuss with the good Doc before we leave" I said with a smile on my face. I think. The silent, gasping expression froze across their faces as they took each other's hands, stood in bewildered astonishment, and with eyes iced in unease, left the room.

Ken and I sat poised in front of Dr. Kobrine seated behind his desk. Pen in hand ready for answers I started checking off my 40 queries one by one as if checking off a grocery list:

1. How long is the surgery? "Won't know until we get in there."

2. What is the recovery time? "Depends upon the outcome."

3. How many of these surgeries have you performed? With a smile upon his face..."Many."

4. How successful have they been? "Very."

5. How long will I be in the hospital? "Depends."

6. Will you shave my head? "Well, we could shave the right side and back leaving a strip in front of your right ear and your hair long on the left so you can comb it over."

   Holy Crap! I'm going to have the balding man comb over!

7. Will I remember it, the surgery, Kenny, my family, my business, my life? "I will do the best I can." Then with an impish grin upon his face he continued, "As one slip of the scalpel and oops there goes college." Then seriously, "You will not have a name file any longer, that's for sure."

8. What would happen if I were still pregnant? "Both you and the baby would die as the hormonal changes would accelerate

the tumor growth by 60% and, being you are already well past the eleventh hour, you would be totally inoperable."

Suddenly in his answer all of our life dreams were annihilated, gone, as if none mattered because we, as we knew us, no longer mattered nor existed.

I know there were other questions prior to that one yet somewhere in the midst of reality it set in through the fog of complete disbelief that this was my life, our life. With Kenny sitting beside me, in this moment, I deflated like a balloon. I broke down in a pool of tears, weeping irrepressibly. The good doc came around to the front of his desk relaxing his tush upon its edge as he folded his long, lanky arms across his solar plexus. His eyes looked through to my heart as he said; "Thank God. I was really beginning to worry about you. Now, we can get real."

Real we did get. Scary real. Statistics: The odds were 80/20 not in my favor of even making it off the table, and an 80% chance of being in a vegetative state for the rest of my life if I did. We were told we were clocking in at the 59th minute of the 11th hour. Kenny shared later that "This was the freakiest thing for me. The slim chance of your coming out of this intact." I do not remember how the consult came to a completion. I am sure something like, 'The front desk will give you surgery date options for you.' I remember Ken and I stood. Ken shook Dr. Kobrine's hand. Maybe I did. We turned and left the room Kenny holding onto my hand as if (and in truth), I would collapse if he didn't. As we entered the reception room, there sat Mom and Dad looking like two frightened kids who had yet to exhale after being told to sit and be quiet in the hallway outside the principal's office. I had never seen my parents, two well-educated, self-assured, grounded in every moment people with the look of controlled terror on their faces. As Kenny walked over to the front desk, I placed a smile on my face walking over to them. They stood as I gently took their hands and asked in a sweet, self-composed manner, "Dad, Mom, would you do us a favor and go get the car? We will be down soon." I could feel every fiber of their being shaking as their bodies turned to leave while their eyes remained glued on me. They turned to looked one more time before they closed the reception room door. And that bald lady is staring at me again.

Meanwhile, I was about to jump out of my skin, or the window, or totally loose it in some form or fashion, I knew not what. So, while Kenny seemed to have things under his control at the front desk, I brushed beside him, placed my hand on his back, and said with pretend ease, as if going out to the garden to pick flowers, "Honey, I am just going into the bathroom for a moment. I will be right out." The look upon his face as he turned was breathlessly endearing. He was doing his very best imitation of, "I've got this. You go ahead."

I heard the door close behind me as I realized I was in one of the tiniest rooms I had ever been in. Kinda like what my inner being, life force, and nature of existence was feeling. I locked the door just in case an innocent intruder or my not knowing what I was going to do. Either way no one need be witness to it. My hands braced the sink. I needed grounding. I stared into the mirror at myself looking through my eyes in deep quietude and inner soul conversation. I tried to figure out if this was really me in the mirror or just an image someone was placing before me that I was to believe was me.

I was about to pass out when I heard myself say; "OK, I can do this. I can do this. But, it's November so... We will wait until after Thanksgiving, and then there's Christmas. Nobody does this, has brain surgery, over the holidays. I can't do that to Kenny nor our families! Then there's New Year's and Oh, Valentine's followed by our Anniversary and then Easter... OK, I can do this... Sometime in the Spring, we'll talk *about it. But then there's Mother's Day and Father's Day...OK, I can do this. Sometime next year after all the important dates are honored. I can do this..."*

I felt I had talked myself into the brave place I needed to be and it was safe to open the bathroom door cause I had it all understood and myself together. Breathe in - Breathe out...I've got this... Door is opening...I'm walking to stand beside my husband, Kenny, and from there I will take over with the scheduling date.

As my body came even with his up against the reception desk, Kenny turned to me and said, "OK, we're set. Your surgery is set for Thursday, November 16th at George Washington University Hospital." Kenny took the first possible surgical date as there was no reason for delay. "What! We can't do that! There's... " And I went into my bathroom logic calendar litany. At which time, as if in unison both Kenny and Cindy Kobrine, Dr. Arthur Kobrine's wife and Office Manager, said, "You cannot wait. It has to be now. We are well past the eleventh hour of the eleventh hour."

In that moment, the bald woman, who had been staring at me, came up wrapping her arms around me, nearly kissing me, saying, "You are going to be alright. I made it through and so will you." I wanted to scream, "Oh My God! Who is this freaky, bald woman hugging me, telling me I am going to be alright?" Every fiber of my being was numb. My facial expression froze in a mini smile of *'Oh Thank You. I feel so much better now.'* I believe Kenny took my hand and led me through the reception room multitudes, into the elevator by way of the beige hallway, into Mom and Dad's car. He held my hand while we traveled through Washington into Maryland, placed my still rigid body into our car and he took control of our drive home from a first for everything. Home from an exceptionally surreal day, that no one would expect their life to be living.

I do not remember at what time of night or if it was that night that I finally exhaled after my silent gasp inward. I do remember I fell into a silent void. I had only nine - 9 - count them, 9 days until I might not be here anymore.

Hold On, Honey

"Dr. Spencer Olson's office. This is Regina. How may I help you?"

"Hello, it's Kenny. I have a surprise for you. I want to take you away. I called Dr. Kobrine and your Dad asking permission to take you on vacation. Dr. Kobrine said, 'If you are going to do it, do it now because there may not be a chance to do so later.' Your Dad said, 'Yes' as well."

"Honey, you are so sweet! This gives me great hope that you believe too that all will be well. After my surgery and recovery, it will be so perfect for us to go away, just us." Just us. What a concept. We had not taken what others would call a vacation in the eight years we had been married."

"No, now, not after surgery, now."

"Honey, I can't just walk out and leave Spencer. I just finished training yet another one of his cutie hires, and she is no way ready to be on her own."

Kenny persisted.

"Seriously! OK, hold on, Honey, I'll go ask Spencer and I'll be right back"

I chuckled inside as I navigated the path holding onto the walls from my front reception desk to my boss's back office. In the office, only Spencer and his wife, Tracy, (yes, Spencer Tracy) knew I was that unsteady. We kept my brain tumor friend on the Q-T (low-down) as symptoms had become quite noticeable. As I took a seat, I knew I was smiling as if about to tell a joke, and this time I would remember the punch line, which, in my opinion, was a doozy.

"Hey, Spencer, Kenny is on the line and wants to know if I can leave on Friday, three days from now, ' cause he wants to take me on vacation before my brain surgery?"

I totally cracked myself up laughing. This was Monday, which would mean we would have only Tuesday, Wednesday, and Thursday before I left the office. Spencer is almost always out of the office on Thursdays, which leaves only two real days, before I would take my leave. This is the business I and Spencer built since his graduation from Palmer Chiropractic College six years ago. I was scheduled to leave two weeks from this day with a good possibility of never returning. The thought of leaving, possibly never to return, in and of itself was enough for me to deal with.

"So, Spence, ain't that a hoot?"

He was looking right at me until he heard my question. Then he looked down at his desk as if studying something important, but I knew better. He didn't even look up when he answered!

"Sure, go ahead."

"What? Did you hear what I asked you, and do you understand the timing involved?"

"Yes. Go ahead."

"OK, ya'll are acting crazy since my diagnosis. I do not know what to do with this."

"Hey, Honey," Spence said, 'Sure, go ahead.' This is crazy, you know. Shouldn't we wait until afterwards and then go?"

Hanging up from my beloved who just wanted to make me feel better, and wonderful and excited about his surprise, I felt a little weird as if maybe all the work I had been doing to convince myself I would make it through might be questionable. With the way folks were acting, maybe this was our last chance in this lifetime for a special time away together.

Friday came. I decided to tell only two of our patients because I did not need people looking at me sad faced as if I was already casket ready with the "Ahh" caught in their throat. Spencer agreed and knowing the two chosen, their positive thought processes would sprinkle prayers upward high into all good possibility land.

The real thoughts, statistics handed to us just days before, had shocked us to our core. I worked really hard at appearing as if I were handling it.

Now, walking as best I could out of my office door Friday evening for what could be my last time, I had a tiny bit of a sinking dead woman walking feeling rushing over me.

There, close enough to take hold of my hand, stood my best friend husband promoting himself as my chauffeur. He had done so for months as the possibility of seizures made driving an unsafe concept for me and anyone else on the road within the state of Maryland.

I gazed into Kenny's eyes through my tears and as he guided me to my waiting chariot, I realized in that moment how tightly he was Holding On, Honey, to me.

Breathe, just breathe...

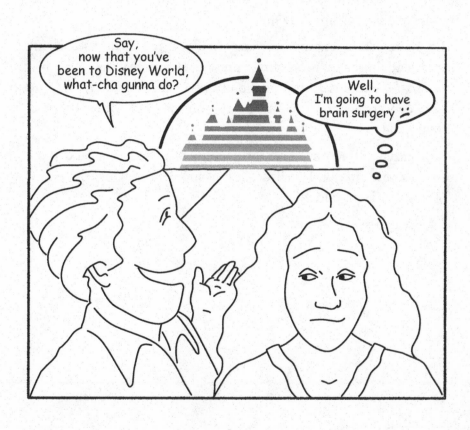

Now That You've Been To Disney World

Kenny took me to Disney World for our "vacation". Yep, the place on earth where dreams come true, supposedly, but as much as we wished, the brain tumor wasn't going away.

Disney World with my beloved, best friend, boyfriend, brain tumor or not, was a dream come true. Kenny cared for me through the pain and unsteadiness as we journeyed. We drove from Maryland as flying with the active tumor was out of the question. Kenny created a Queen's Throne for me in the van with pillows and bean bags. He watched over me as much as he checked out the roads we were traveling. Left eye on roads. Right eye on me.

Once inside the Magic Kingdom, I admit it, just like a seven-year young little girl, I cried when I stood in front of Cinderella's Castle, waiting for Tinker Bell to fly out and overhead any moment. No one had a better eye-catching panorama than I did. All three days and into the nights, through parades, strolls and destination locations I was seeing the world, both ours and Disney's from up top Kenny's shoulders. I was, we were, just one of the kids in our own little kid grown-up world.

Of course, we rode the One World little kid coaster singing along to "It's A Small World After All." We stood in line for at least forty-five minutes to catch the ride on Space Mountain with its loop-de'-loops, upside down turns, and the straight down dive into middle earth. What was I doing in this line? I don't do rides! I don't even do Ferris wheels at carnivals. You will be hard pressed to get me on a merry-go-round in your hometown park. Kenny was little boy excited and really wanted me to go with him. Meanwhile I'm thinking *I have just as much a chance of dying or coming out in a vegetative state on that crazy ass ride as I do from my brain tumor.* Hmmmm....Choices.

Oh, thank you, 6 pound, 8 ounce Baby Jesus, there's a sign clearly stating the Rules and Regulations upon boarding this train.... "Blah, Blah, Blah...If you have seizures...Blah, Blah, Blah...If you stand less than 5 feet...Blah, Blah, Blah..." We were three into being the next to ascend into madness. "Kenny, Look, Honey, I can't go!" I pointed to the sign with my faux sad face, lips in a frown, which by no means fooled the man. "OK, we won't go." "No, you go, I'll meet you on the other side in Europe." This ride plummeted over every continent of planet earth from outer space. I would need to seek out the end point but, hey, that's better than creating my own. "Go! Go!", I said. And he did. Standing amidst the crowd, watching him board, I was praying to God for his safe return this side of life. I had no idea how long the ride was. "Seven minutes" the conductor said. OK, I have seven minutes to navigate my way to Europe through what could be a bizarre, freaky world. I was not up for a multitude of pressing throngs and oversized cartoon characters, unless, of course, Dopey came along with me. That would be kinda OK.

I heard myself telepathically sending messages to Kenny from inside my head; *I'm here. It's been 10 minutes. Where are you?* Keep calm, eyes bright, breathe and walk on through miles of Disney World as if you know where you are. Just keep walking, just keep walking, just keep walking...It's been an hour...Ooh, a "Do Not Enter" sign. Secret... If you want to find Kenny in an unfamiliar place anywhere in all of the world, look for the "Do Not Enter" sign. Of course, me, being the good girl, I did not enter. I did however wait outside until the door opened and Kenny re-entered my fairytale world. Big Hugs, Big Exhales. "When I didn't see you in Italy, I thought, I'll go in here for a few minute" Kenny said. *Yea...*

Meanwhile, there was much more to explore. The days and nights were full of wonder, joyful happiness, sensational magic and worlds away from MRI scans, doctors, wills, funeral planning and the idea of anyone taking a knife to my head.

We ate ice cream, funnel cakes, and pizza. We held conversations with Mickey and Minnie and a Princess or two. Kenny had quite the chat with Goofy. We walked until I could no longer, then we got a wheelchair. We laughed and played and cried knowing this could be our last revelry before the intense drama begins, but we did not say it aloud. I remember at one-point riding high a'top Kenny's shoulders strolling behind an elderly couple holding hands walking slower than pleased the crowd. No words were necessary. We stopped and held each other through our weeping as we knew we were them in our youth. Every now and then reality gently showed itself through the mist of make believe.

We went to every exhibition and World this and World that including Epcot Center with the Michael Jackson Thriller experience. Then it appeared, a ride within a seated auditorium that supposedly shrunk you down so that you could ride through the human body, exploring every cell and organ including the brain. What? I had to be there. No ups and downs just imagination. I can do that. We stood in line until a small uniformed guy came over and asked, "Are you sure about being shrunk down to size?" "Absolutely." Seriously, imagination, I can do that. Staying seated in a nailed in place chair on a cement auditorium floor while viewing body systems like the brain. I can do that. "Kenny, I've got to see this. There may be something I need to know." So, staffer of imagination, waved a wand over us leading us into the theater to our seats on the end, third row. I was excited. A ride in a big room, no movement and I might learn something. Go!

Ahhh, wait a minute...Why are we clicking into seat belts? "Kenny, if I start to go out, I'll just put my head down between my knees. Stay with me." "No problem. It's just a movie." Lights dimmed.

The front seat of a little roller coaster appeared on the screen as if we were sitting in it. *I'm OK, it's just a picture*, I thought to myself. Suddenly my chair was no longer nailed to the cement floor but raising and damn, it's tipping right, left, front, back as we travel through the blood system from the heart into I haven't a clue what body part because I am about to pass out. Quick head down between knees, hands flat on cement floor. I'll just stay here and listen and learn but, holy crap, this is a roller coaster ride without the bugs in your teeth.

Kenny's reassuring hand was on my back. "It'll be over soon Honey, hang in." Sooner than we thought, because suddenly in unison everybody's chairs came to an air-whooshing, hydraulic release as they settled back into the position of start. The lights came on, the screen went blank, and a door hidden within the inside body mural on the wall opened. A stern looking, khaki-clothed man looked right at me and pointed his finger saying; "YOU, OUT!"

I sat up straighter than I knew was possible since third grade Catholic parochial school being called out for the wades of toilet paper on the ceiling in the boys' bathroom, which by the way I did not do. I taught them how, but I did not do it. While pointing to my chest I asked without words; "Me?" "YES, YOU! OUT!" Damn, I really wanted to do this. What if there's something I need to know in here before my brain surgery and I'm going to miss it? "Go ahead, Honey. Stay right outside the door. I'll check it out for anything we may need to know and be right out."

Crap, there I go again, into multitudes of I don't know you people. Big inhale...Big exhale...I stood up and thought, *OK, I am going to use this opportunity to possibly help others*. I stood, turned to the numerous rows of folks behind our third-row seating and said; "I am your excuse. If anyone else wants out, follow me." I headed toward the door on the right as did six other women right behind me. The door shut behind us. I'm staying right here. All six of us slinked down the walls of the hall onto the floor where it was steady and we could feel secure in the world again, at least this part of Disney World. I heard it over and over again; "Thank You for being my way out." "Hey, anything I can do."

Then it came. The time where we would have to leave this enchantment hopeful that we could take some of its supernatural spell and fairy dust back with us. Loudspeaker voices announcing last call, exit through the gate to your left, as lights began to dim and super-sized characters of our childhood slowly disappeared. *I didn't know there was a door in that tree.* There was a crushing pack of humanity all leaving through the same egress. Once again Kenny saved me by the gymnastics of riding on his shoulder. As everyone leaves through this portal there is a large marine tank, in which dolphins resided. We were in the back of the herd, yet I heard a calling. A calling I had to answer. "Kenny, I've got to be there." We pushed our way through the crowd up to the glass wall dividing water species and earthling. People were smacking the water top with the flattened edge of their palms. I could barely breath, there was such a senseless crude force in their actions. I watched the beautiful aqua dancers each becoming more and more understandably upset with the continuous drumming of water and the reverberations felt within their heads and hearts. There were eight dolphins and with every circling they drew further and further away from the crazy mortals clinging closer and closer to the inside centered column swimming round and round, faster and faster. How could this be? Are they treated this way every night? Why would Disney people design them at the exit? This was awful. I felt their fear. I needed to ask their forgiveness. And should one touch me, forever I would be grateful as this may be the last time anything like that would happen in my existence on earth.

I closed my eyes. I placed my hand first on top on the water. No movement, just hand, just thoughts of forgiveness. People totally oblivious to the wonder amidst them started pushing by us anxious to heed the automated bullhorn instructions to exit. Eyes still closed, I extended my left hand further into the depths of their marine home. I could feel a calmness blanketing my new friends. Although I could perceive it within my heart, I opened my eyes in time, before being rushed out of the park, to see the captives slowing their flowing pace. Just in that moment one swam right under my left hand, slowly, purposefully, feeling like the most magnificent Angel with wet silk skin. He chose to touch me in loving gratitude. He knew this may be my last chance ever this time on earth to experience what they have to give to humans. Ecstasy filled every cell of my being overflowing and connecting his soul with mine. The moment of non-verbal language between species lasted a long enough lifetime from his spiritual perspective. This exquisitely elegant sleek creature, as his tail completed his final touch into my world, turned and looked deeply into my eyes transmitting the thought of *Peace be with you*. Smiling he softly faded into the inner circle of his family. This was a Beloved God Moment. It is one of the most overflowing gratitude moments of my life that, to this day, I can re-feel in every cell of my body. Ken held me as I turned into his chest and wept.

We walked quietly toward our vehicle holding tightly to each other's hands amidst the noisy night crowd. There was nothing further to say as we had experienced the joy of momentary relief from the reality we were walking back into. We settled into our seats and just as Kenny started to turn the key in the ignition, an impish smirk came across his face as he ask the Super Bowl Winners question, but this time with a twist, "Now that you've been to Disney World, whatcha gonna do?" I chimed right in with, "I'm gonna have Brain Surgery!"

My Last Monday...Tuesday ...Wednesday...
Ever In This Lifetime

It just dawned on me...What if this is the last Monday I will ever live here on what I know as earth? It's just the start of the work week as we know it and yet by Thursday I may be gone. That's only a few days from now. What if tomorrow is my last Tuesday? Usually on Tuesdays I clean the bathroom and go on with my day from there.

I don't know, do they have bathrooms in Heaven? Do they clean them on Tuesdays? Do they have Tuesdays? Do they have to go to the bathroom in Heaven? I certainly wouldn't think so. It just seems so below a Heavenly thing to have to do, but, then again, God did design this body. But I won't have this body.

What if Wednesday is my last Wednesday? How does one knowingly spend their last Wednesday? Their last Day?

What if this is my last Monday, my last Tuesday, my last Wednesday to look at Kenny's face? Will his face look different from Heaven?

I am not sure how to do this. Nobody said anything about knowing this may be your last Monday or any day of the week.

If I just sit and contemplate the very fact that this may be true, it seems to be a colossal waste of time, time which is literally and possibly ticking away from me. Then again, it's not like I have a huge bucket list. I'm not old enough to have a bucket list. There is nothing I need to do to feel complete. I just am.

Is "Just am" good enough, if this is my last Monday?

Little Story - Big Memory

My Button Collection

I wrote my will the night before going into the hospital. I wrote it on a yellow loose-leaf, lined piece of paper and signed it. I wanted Kenny to have first choice of everything, I asked him, "It matters most to me what you want before anyone else. What would you like left from me?"

He looked over with serenity in his eyes and answered, "I want your button collection." I am not sure how long I stared while holding my breath. I didn't even know he knew I had a button collection. "It gives you such joy. I want your button collection. But it will still be here when you get home."

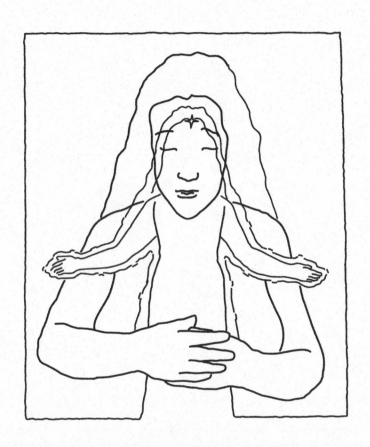

Jesus, Elizabeth, and Me

Chapter Two

In The Hospital Well Past The Eleventh Hour Navigating The Land Of Uncertainty

Jesus, Elizabeth and Me
November 16, 1989

The 5:30 early morning wake-up for a 7:00 am surgery timeline is a memory fog interspersed with reality. *Please don't unwrap me from the safety of Kenny's bedded embrace.* I remember being assisted onto a gurney, Kenny by my side. I remember my eyes were wide, my heart pounding, my life energy caught in my upper arms, my breath a prisoner in my upper chest and throat, and every sense that is physical numbingly on hyper alert.

I remember the sound from the wheel's wobble of the gurney turning under my body on the hospital laminate floor as we traveled toward the unknown, Kenny by my side. I laid there taken captive, strapped in, able to look only where my detained eyes were allowed to look from a point of arrest. Light after long fluorescent ceiling light marked our journey. The world had been turned upside down mimicking the white lines on a highway in darkened hours of night. Glimpses of hospital scenery, photos on the walls honoring the lineage of doctors who had toured the hall long before my nomadic sojourn, nurses paused in the hallway as if waiting for the light to change and their turn to pass. I heard whispered chatter yet could not make out what anyone was saying as if they were far away in a rolled tube of animation reverberating much like what I imagine the first phone call ever made through can and wire might have sound like.

Then the door, the dividing door of life as I, as we, knew it up and to this point and what life would and will be, if there is to be, on the other side. I had watched Kenny's face behind the crown of my head since the moment he had to leave my side letting go of my hand giving up his sacred space to the attendant in charge of navigation. Kenny's face, his handsome, I love you face, eyes wide, the laugh lines I first noticed in the halls of school that drew me to his heart, now with an expression, if it were to be called an expression, I had never seen before. It was a mix of fear, I am being courageous for you, I am holding my own because if I don't, who will. There was a longing showing through his soul, a longing that this was not real and if it really were that we were already on the other side of this momentary millennium of time and all was well.

For me from where I lay, I studied every line of his face capturing and freezing it in my forever memory bank never to be unlocked until the kiss of time told me it was safe to come out again because he would be there to catch me as I fall out of the pages of this story being told about us. Now or in another lifetime I wanted to recognize those eyes, and the details of art written through life across his face. His compassionate eyes, his dark silk hair and beard, his mouth with the most perfect curves. I was memorizing, collecting every memory of his face thinking, *This may be it, the last time I ever see his face, him, in this lifetime from this side of living. What if I do come back not able to express, I'M HERE, so people know that I AM HERE? I want from the other side of that invisible contained wall to know, to recognize, his face so that from there, in my own little mist of a world, he is still there in his.*

Fear building, the moment came, I had to let go of his hand for the last time as the gurney garcon pushed our life through what would become the dividing line double doors. My eyes watched as his body figure became thinner and thinner as the door's center groove closed in between us.

I was now on my own with a barrage of people I did not know. I remember trying to smile as if to please those moving me from the wheeled flat plate to the cold covered table in the OR set for my surgery. My surgery...What was I doing here? How did this happen? Why did it have to be our, my reality? Was this reality or had I slipped into another dimension through a very thin wrinkle between worlds? Was there an escape to be taken if I but pushed, investigated, surveyed, wandered with hope for another preferred fantasy?

Nope, it's happening, really happening all around and through me. I am doing my best to appear as if I am in complete control of all my senses and possibly everyone else's. One thing I am not doing is letting go. I know I am sitting on the edge of what will become my lie down place for the next, I haven't a clue how long. I know there is a person standing in front of me between my dangling legs, telling me what is okay to tell me about what is about to happen and that I am just fine. I know I am looking at her and probably have that thin line upward lip on my face as if I appear to be hearing her, so she feels better about what is to happen. I also know I am not taking anything she is saying into my realm as if there were a gauzy wall of dimensional shift between us. There are mortal citizens of the OR, the myriad of souls that make it run smoothly, in the background like all the humans one sees in the background of a subway scene. You know they are there but what they are doing there is beyond your need to know. I know there are people, I am sure very kind people, behind me touching my head, talking about my head, moving my hair and where they will shave it in reference to where my cranium will be cut. They are drawing lines with their fingers either in the air or smack up against my skull. It's hard to tell because everything is becoming everything right now and I am not sure I am going to survive this moment because my heart is beating so intensely hard I literally can see my chest move in and out with every beating thump and with every beat and every outward thrust I'm thinking, *I'm not going to die of a brain tumor, I'm going to die of a heart attack! I can't breathe! God! Jesus! Please Elizabeth! I Can't Breathe! Help Me!*

Help Me... Help Me... Help Me softly and sweetly became an echo as all faded away into a gray mist. There was no operating room. There were no people. There were no walls. There was No Thing. There was standing in front of me my Savior, my Master-Teacher of Angels and Humanity, my Spiritual Brother, my Jesus and my Guardian Angel, Elizabeth as ONE yet their separate Selves. In the immediacy of life lived, un-lived and yet to be, I was enveloped into the very essence of Peace. I could smell it, feel it, taste it, I, with Them, was IT. They stood in a Glow of Light embracing every cell of existence including my own. They together smiled with outstretched arms bringing me into Their tranquil embrace in a place of no time and no mortal circumstance. I was with Them, in the purity of safety, wellness and all possibility of what matters and no matter. I was smiling basking in God Joy. There were no words in our intercourse, yet all was perfectly understood.

I am Okay, if I die today. I am Okay, if I become in a vegetative state. And You know what I want. I am asking You please if I die, if I become in a vegetative state, to take good care of Kenny. That's all. And You know what I want. Thank You. Thank You for being here with me always.

Their arms still outstretched embracing my being, They together as One yet Their single selves, Elizabeth behind and within Jesus's beating heart, the Light bathing me in the truth of believable bliss of all knowing with no need to understand nor comprehend. They touched me everywhere far beyond what is a created body in a living world. We were In Love, Jesus, Elizabeth and Me and all was well.

I laid down and closed my eyes. I remember the sound of the saw. I remember the numbed touch.

It's Okay, if I die today. It's Okay if I become in a vegetative state.

And You know what I want. Thank You. Amen.

And in the silence of an inner world comforted by my celestial visitors amidst the structured chaos of the operating room, our three voices harmonized in prayer. The prayer I had been saying two, three, five times and more daily since the three days after the long nights before, studying every line, integrating its personal message of survival this lifetime and beyond. Together....

The LORD is my shepherd; I shall not want.

He makes me to lie down in green pastures

He leads me beside the still waters.

He restores my soul

He leads me in the paths of righteousness for His name's sake

Yea, though I walk through the valley of the shadow of death

I will fear no evil

For You are with me

Your rod and Your staff they comfort me.

You prepare a table before me in the presence of my enemies

You anoint my head with oil

My cup runs over.

Surely goodness and mercy shall follow me

all the days of my life

And I will dwell in the house of the LORD forever.

Psalm 23

Rumor Has It
Part I
Two Docs Two Dads Hush Accord

Rumor has it my Dad was thrown out of the Operating Room where I lay being readied for a craniotomy. I'd say I wasn't there being I have no memory of the moment, but I was there. I was just really out of it, quite literally, out of it, the plan and consciousness.

Evidently my Dad, Dr. Alfred John Suraci, a Reconstructive Surgeon along with one of the attending neurosurgeons had come to an understanding I call The Two Docs - Two Dads Hush Accord. Rumor has it, went something like this: Dad wanted to be in the OR with me even though being a Doc he was well aware of the medical profession's unspoken notion having a family member in the OR during a surgery is most assuredly not the best idea in the world. Still he really wanted to be there. From a daughter's point of view, it is a sweet gesture even though this daughter was totally unaware of the scheme. I guess they figured the less folks who knew of their stealth plan the less likely for it to be foiled. I'm thinking from the officiating surgeon's point of view it could be rather nerve racking to have the doctor dad breathing over your shoulder. But docs are gods in their fields so at least that day the gods were in alignment. I suspect Dad thought he could get away with it being his last name was different from mine so who would know. I'm guessing Dad came in after I was laid out flat as I have no memory of his being present. If I had been even a little bit more awake, I would remember those doting eyes peeking out over the surgical mask. Anyway after Dad was suited up and in, rumor has it somebody got wind of the fact that Doc Suraci was the patient's Dad and somehow or another he was asked to leave the arena for the very reasoning it's really not a good idea to have the dad of the daughter about to have her head sawed open in the same room no matter how detached that last semester of med school taught one to be.

I can only imagine Dad's inner outrage, heartfelt disappointment and outer dismay. My Dad being asked to leave anywhere would be paramount in and of itself and certainly this was a new and un-welcomed experience in his book. My Dad invented control, authority and supremacy in the medical field. He was King Control. Somehow, I am sure, in his mind, if he were at least a silent "observer" in the room he had some command over the situation in his heart as his daughter was having brain surgery. Not being in the Operating Room the way he wanted left him out of the loop, out of power. If there was one position my Father had a lesser idea of how to handle, it was the personal life out of control jurisdiction region. He not only left the OR, he left the hospital.

When I heard my Mom's compelling expression of this gagged rumor of my Dad being thrown out of the OR, and leaving the hospital without even saying "Got to go" to my Mom, I could not help but think, *Hello! Wife! Mother of Daughter having brain surgery is in the family waiting room! She may want/need your support.* Seriously, Dad left Mom to pace the floor there on her own. When I say on her own, I do not mean alone, as both Kenny and Pattie were there running their own paces right along with her. But meanwhile her husband, the other half of making this grown baby was not.

My heart went out to my Dad as I heard about the near perfect masquerade. He pretended to be this man, who happened to be a doctor, who just wanted to see a brain surgery but in reality, he, this father-doctor wanted to be as close to his daughter's beating heart as he possibly could because it just may stop.

How deeply endearing was that silently screaming heartfelt bravery. Dad being in the OR was his prayer in action and when that was not a possibility, he needed a distraction, the distraction of taking care of his own patients of the day. He could not carry the same strength his wife, the mother of their child, was bearing, being present far from the side of their daughter. When his higher plan failed, he could not embrace the scare and knowing my Dad, having cleared his day from his surgical endeavors, more than likely he went into church to pray. Pray a Father's prayer of Love, Please and Thank You before he went off to take care of other parent's sons and daughters. Rumor Has It, that's what Doc-Dad's do.

Rumor Has It
Part II
Out Of The Mouth Of A Different Kinda Babe

Anesthesia can make you silly and having brain surgery might just make you say things you wouldn't normally say, especially out loud in, how you say, mixed company. Still in first recovery, rumor has it, crazy waking words came out of my mouth as folks waited with bated breath for me to come back to this life after six hours plus of brain surgery and the day is now moving into the night. Rumor has it, as I opened my medically induced sleeping eyes, gazing into Kenny's, the first words out of my slipstreamed mouth were, "Climb on up here and do me, Big Boy." Seriously! So not like me! At least that's what Kenny and Pattie told me I said. Way out of range of my way of expressing myself. My take is those present who witnessed this totally not like me moment, Kenny, Pattie and the recovery nurse, either collaborated in these loose lips testimony or someone played with the potty mouth part of my brain while in there earlier in the day. I'd like to say I wasn't there but, either way as I fell right back into a sedative sleep, they all had a startling good laugh and actually do to this day when the subject comes back round.

Twenty minutes later, Kenny and Pattie were still by my side with nurse close by. Rumor has it, I stirred momentarily in a sobbing surge, "Honey, we won't be able to do it for a really long time. I just had brain surgery." Seriously, what's with all the whoopee on my mind? Who went where in there and did what? Again, after my new way of letting it all hang out, I fell right back into a deep siesta. Rumor has it and as it has been threatened, you're coming out of anesthesia waking words may outlive you being spoken as a sweet little memory at your funeral one day long time from now.

Eyes closed, laying still, next thing I heard was my Mother's voice, "Kenny, it's 8:30. We should let her rest. You need your rest. Her Father is waiting out in the car and we should go." *I heard that! That's just crazy talk! My Father is leaving without coming in to say good night to me! Hello! Daughter! Brain Surgery!* Later Mom told me my way of expressing my outrage went something like; "I just had brain surgery! You tell Dad to get his butt in here and kiss me good-night!" Holy Crap! I have never spoken like that to either of my parents! Are we sure I didn't have a mouth-ectomy while under some funny gas? I said Dad and butt in the same sentence and got away with it! What seemed only moments later, I do remember through slit eye view Kenny and Dad standing beside me as I laid working to wake. Dad had that funny smirk on his face, the one with the upside-down smile. His hand was on my shoulder, I heard him say through my gauzed ears; "I got my butt in here to say good-night. Good-Night." He kissed my forehead before turning to leave, "Nightie Night" I heard him whisper with a smile. I was out with a twinkle.

In this Recovery Room they had a big, really big ass, oops potty mouth word I don't usually say out loud, clock on the wall facing the foot of my gurney. I suppose that was to give patients comfort in that if you see a clock you must be rousing from your ordeal here on earth because rumor has it they don't bother with time on the other side. Here on earth they don't add the day of the week and it's coordinating color of jello until you are up settled in your appointed room. Too much information is just that. At this point of step-down recovery, they are working with you on a need to know only scenario.

Well, there I was hours later in a momentary eye opening. I do remember it was 11:00 pm as there was that big ass, oops there's that word again, clock staring right back at me. I swear it smiled.

Everyone I knew was gone from sight except the dedicated recovery nurse still on shift. I remember her face, her hair, her smile, her scrubs as she went about her duties.

They are necessary duties as much for the one coming back into this worldly state of mind as they are for those making sure you are coming back into this worldly state of mind. It's just a little crazy how as the anesthesia is working its way out of you finally you are getting another kind of sleep, good heavy sleep, necessary, good, heavy sleep for recovery but I think that scares them so they just happen to wake you a little bit now and then as they take your vitals. "Oh, you're awake" they say. Like they didn't know that big ass needle prick wouldn't animate the living dead. It's their 'Not gonna die on my shift' training.

In that moment of blood pressure pumping blood to the brain, I guess, I realized the time and the day, 11:00 pm on a Thursday night. Pretty amazing after brain surgery only half a day earlier. The nurse still by my side, I voiced my disappointment when I realized; "Oh crap! I missed Hill Street Blues!" The nurse's bewildered facial expression said it all; "Seriously, this is what's important to you right now?" No... No, not really...Sleep...Sleep good...Snooze...I'm out.

The Pattie Kiss
"Doctor! Doctor! My Brain Hurts"

My baby sister Pattie is a funny girl. Sometimes she's funny just to be funny. Sometimes she's funny to make someone else feel better. Sometimes she's funny so she can handle a situation, a moment in time that is less comfortable than she would like it to be. Sometimes she's funny when she wants you to hear something that's really not funny, but she seriously wants to get your attention. There were occasions during my brain tumor surgery and recovery she was employing all four tactics at once with an ease that would make late night comic writers envious.

Evidently there was this line from the Monty Python Flying Circus TV Series skit entitled "Doctor! Doctor! My Brain Hurts." At that point and time, I had yet to see it, I think. I had to ask Kenny as TV and movie-like memory is a curious thing with me. Kenny and I have a code when I am not remembering something. It goes like this: BBS = Before Brain Surgery and ABS = After Brain Surgery. Movies still are a question mark unless a movie really grabs me for one reason or another, such as the infamous phrase from the movie *Love Story* — BBS, "Love means never having to say you're sorry." Seriously? Really? Oh, Please.

This next one is a real movie memory maker for me. One that will never be forgotten because it happened to me before the movie was ever made. The scene in the movie *Phenomenon* — ABS, where John Travolta's character is hit and knocked down by the oncoming ginormous brilliance in a flash of light. He was in the middle of the street. I was at Bob's Big Boy in Annapolis, Maryland.

Or how 'bout a scene, like the one where Meg Ryan's doctor character is riding her bike, arms extended, head thrown back in total surrender for the first time ever since childhood, heart totally peeled for all the world to viscerally caress, in a definite favorite movie of mine, *City of Angels* — ABS. You know the scene, the one that screams, Holy Crap, she's going to die!

Or when the sweet, bedtime chignon coifed white haired old lady climbs up the boat railings of the *Titanic* — ABS, to drop the larger than life cobalt gem into the depths of the heart of the ocean. It wasn't the gem that seized that moment for me. It was the little old ladies' hands. They reminded me of my Mom's. Not that my Mom was ever a little old lady 'cause she wasn't, but the hands, her hands, were so beautiful and because of that clip I totally lost it in the movie theatre before any Titanic tragedy had floated into our spectator minds. Thus, the creation of BBS and ABS.

The Monty Python thing, I wasn't so sure. Come to find out, I had yet to see it. Now that I have, I totally understand why Pattie and our friend, Rick, who happened to be an Emergency Room nurse at GW, on numerous occasions came in the room stiff board bodied, steel cold eyes, wearing corner twisted hankies on their heads, quietly hospital screaming in British accents, "Doctor! Doctor! My Brain Hurts!" Pattie on the other hand, saw the show, loved it and had integrated it into her existence as a lifesaving nurse. There we were sitting together. Me tucked under sterile covers as she sat on top of the sheets of my bed, 5th floor, GW University Hospital. She was just so totally joy filled I was alive that every cell of her little body exuded the declaration right into my heart. She was saying funny things, I am sure, although often at that point of recovery, I would slip in and out of consciousness. Often, she stayed for hours on end. I knew that, as when I would wake from one of my eye closing napping states of mind, she would still be there. I guess she could have slipped out in-between but when would she know to come back and be sitting there when I wake?

One evening, probably late night, as she was getting ready to leave, she came over to the right side of my bed, donning the ever present four corner buckled head tissue, again giving great credence to the MP "Doctor! Doctor! My Brain Hurts!". She opened her purse, took out her cosmetic case, slathered her lips before leaving for the snow layered earthly exterior, leaned over the don't fall out of your bed bars and kissed my turban wrapped head, right side temporal where the tumor used to be. Pulling back there was the Pattie twinkle of, "I crack myself up" in her eyes with matching Dad smirk as she turned and took her leave.

Meanwhile, after her departure, nurse after nurse came running into my room with a slight gasp of breath in their throat. I thought, *"What nurse speak revelation did Pattie leave the Nursing Post that each attendant seems highly vigilant in my care all night, all day?"* Once they touched the right temporal side of my turban, they exhaled in great relief leaving the room with a slight shake of their head. I thought, *I'm new here. I'm not sure what they are doing but I'm glad they are doing it in my care.* Finally, Claudette! Oh goody! I get to see Nurse Claudette! Oops! She has that same strangely alarmed look on her face running toward me touching my head. I felt her exhale over my skull. "Who did that to you?" she asked in her Heavenly Havana accent. "Who did what"? "Who kissed you in bright fire engine red lipstick?" "Ohhh... Ahhh! That would be my baby sister, Pattie." "Well, from outside in the hall, it looks like you have a bleed through your turban. That's not a good sign. Isn't she a nurse? She should know better." And with a similar Nurse Pattie twinkle in her eye and a giggle in her voice, she left the room.

Ahhh, I get it. Pattie didn't have to say anything out loud to the Florence Nightingales at the Nurse's Station. She stealth coded; "Take good care of my sister while I'm not here to do so."

"Doctor! Doctor! My Brain Hurts!" And my baby sister Nurse Pattie, is a seriously funny girl!

Fully Alive
Lady Lost Spirit Found

"So, Good Morning. How are you feeling?", his cheery voice asked as he began to fuss over my many wire attachments coming from and going to where I hadn't a clue. He was tall, I think. Well, from where I sat braced in the high railing bed, he was. Tall, dark, near black curly hair, slender build, and an amazingly joyful smile upon his very white face, Lee was my nurse in ICU and I was ever so proud of myself remembering his name. I was working very hard to do so, remember names that is. I had been told prior to surgery that due to the tumor's placement in my brain and the surgery excision more than likely my name memory file along with other personal filing systems in my brain would be removed. As Doc Kobrine said; "If I'm not careful, oops, there goes college." So, I had set my mind to doing my very best to remember all the nurses' names who cared for me in the hospital. To date I still remember Lee and Claudette's facial features and expressions, their bodies, and the clothes they wore as well. They were so kind and compassionate. Lee even came to visit with me the morning of the day of my release home.

Lee continued to do his nursing thing tied up with my wrapped turban, which I was unaware of wearing at the time. "Lee, what is the big, clumpy thing behind my head?" Whenever I lightly leaned my head upon the pillow buttress, I could tell the back of my head was not touching it. I could feel something between me and the soft spot. "That's a drainage bag." I need know no more.

She started screaming again, and the quiet, half lite grey dungeon air was cut with a shrill. My gurney was closest to the door of the right-hand side of ICU. Hers was by the shaded window, polar opposite, same side of the room, to my right. She screamed a lot. "Where am I? Why do you keep asking me those questions? What's happening?" Then just screams. Desperate, fearful, horrible shrieks. Her wailing once again alerted Lee who was tucking something into the back of my head. "I'll be back. Let me go see if I can be of any help." "What's wrong?" "She had brain surgery too." I fell into a place of even more silence so as to be able to hear beyond her inarticulate communication.

Her eerie howls continued and while I could not hear specifically what others were saying, asking or talking about, I could hear the gentle tone in their voices. Part of the ICU nurses' job was to check in with us every hour with a barrage of questions. Questions that may appear simplistic to anyone on the street, but we were not on the street and had not been for a while. "What day is it? Who is the President? What is your name? What is your husband's name? Do you know where you are? How many fingers am I holding up? Do you know what has happened to you" Once I caught on I wanted to play. Question: What day is it? "What color is the jello?" I need answer only once. You can tell what day it is in the hospital by the color of the daily jello bowl. Look out Friday as the dessert menu is brimming with the tie-dye jello assortment of Sunday through Thursday. I must admit, my first President answer was a bit off being it was 1989 and Eisenhower had been long gone from the White House grounds.

"Ken, his name is Kenny." I said with breathless gratitude and a smile. Ken's nightmare, should I live, was I would not know who he was, who we were. He feared our life would have been erased from my memory.

The door to the left of the bottom end of my bed opened, which in and of itself was a rarity as this was the ICU. As a man passed the foot of my bed, I heard her scream; "Stop asking me, what is my husband's name! Stop telling me I am married! I am not married! I have no husband!" My eyes met his soul just as it began to drop out from his chest onto the floor. Oh my God, the shattering of his heart was palatable. The wreckage slowed his foot's pace as he grabbed for my bed's support railing.

For three days and three long, lonely nights she screamed. Her terror shattered the intersection paths of the hallway and sent shivers through the spaces of every corner and circular margin around and within me as if boring through my skin. I wished I could walk. I wished I could walk into her room, slip into the bed beside her and hold her and somehow magically she would be calm, breathing in the rhythm of her new life post craniotomy. I wished she was accepting who she is now in peace and feeling the euphoric bliss I was experiencing even as I too was attached to a back of the head drainage bag. Every scream grabbed my heart and threw it up against the wall spilling something, I knew not what. "Is she going to be okay?" I would ask every nurse who was with me at the time of her feral vocal expressions. "We hope so", was the usual reply.

Three days post our roommate sharing of ICU, I watched from my up against the wall hallway IV shuffle as her husband, head down, heart and soul heavy, slowly pushed the door to his wife's hospital room open. He disappeared into the shriek of: "Who are You? Get out of here! You don't belong in here!". He obviously stayed. He obviously tried to be okay. He obviously loved her.

Monday evening there were no more fearful screams, no more bellows of terror. The halls, the walls, the light fixtures, the air was quiet. I was so hopeful she had been reunited with herself, her husband.

The twilight nurse shift had just begun. "Is she okay?" "Honey, she died this afternoon." "What? Why?" This was all before HIPPA when you could have a compassionate conversation concerning people you did not know but clearly had shared life together. "We do not know why. She just died. She had an 90% chance of making it and she just seemed to give up and died." Had she scared herself to death?

I am not quite sure how long I held my breath but by the time I did exhale, my respiration needed CPR. Ken held me for hours of releasing tears. Was I ever going to understand how it was that she had a 90% chance of living and I had less than a 20% chance of making it off the table, an 80% chance of being in a vegetative state if I did? Yet there I was alive and becoming well while she died not even remembering her husband who loved her so dearly and deeply.

How does this happen? Why does this happen? What does it mean? Why was I alive and she's dead? Was I worthy of such a truth? What must I do to become worthy? I was adding to the excruciating pain already existing in my head from surgery with my turbulent tears and spiritually esoteric questions. Could I sleep? Could I stay awake long enough to grasp even an inkling of comprehension of what just happened? It never occurred to me to give up. Why did she?

For years this reality haunted me until I woke to the faithfulness that she, this woman whom I have never met face to face, the woman in ICU, 3 beds to the right of mine and just 3 doors down on the opposite side of the Neurosurgery Fifth Floor hall, this woman who had a 90% chance of survival but died, is but one of my Inspirations, one of my Teachers, Guiding Lights, Muse, Impulses, Artist of Reality, creating in me my purposeful, ethical integrities of living my authentic life as consciously aware as possible at all times so as to miss out on nothing that is truly of any importance. Realizing there is so little that is truly important and to that which is, pay attention, Fully Alive.

The Op Report

It was Monday night and we were sitting, talking and giggling as if we were at a girlie slumber party versus the truth of Room 525 Fifth Floor Neurosurgery Department in GWU Hospital Center. Me, slipped between bed linens looking as if I belonged to the sheets being the turban wrapped around my broken stitched head fashionably accessorized the matching sterile white bedcovers, while baby sister Nurse Pattie and one of her BFF's at the time Nurse Doris were hanging out in chairs situated close to my cot on wheels. The TV was on as I remember the background noise although I haven't a clue as to what show was running in its usual November 1989 Monday night lineup. Pattie and Doris were really good friends. They both worked at Providence Hospital in DC although in different departments. Pattie in NEO-Natal ICU with babies so tiny they fit in the palm of your hand and Doris with the big babies in need down in the ER. They socialized together; parties, movies, shopping or just hung out at Pattie's townhouse in Greenbelt. They shared lots of life together. They were the female version of Steve Martin and Dan Aykroyd's "Two Wild and Crazy Kinda" Gals. So, it was Doris was sharing my life like a super plus tag-along sister. They were laughing and carrying on as was their usual for hours as I came in and out of consciousness. I do not remember any part of any whole conversation.

I was half awake and probably drooling when a nurse came in the room directing her eyes, motion forward and no-nonsense nurse to nurse announcement to Pattie; "I've got it! The Operative Report! Here it is!" Pattie quickly stood and leaped forward in one swift simultaneous motion taking the envelope with a grasp of intensity. Her eyes widened, her lips pursed, and she seemed to be holding her breath as if the next exhale would be birthed through whatever was hidden within the stationary envelope. As if practiced under synchronous

Olympian trials both Pattie and Doris plunked themselves onto my bunk and the linen went whoosh. Pattie climbed in next to my left side as if she were going to read me a bedtime story while Doris butted up to the left side of my feet, her hands gently resting upon them. "It's your Operative Report. I asked for a copy and have been waiting for it." She held it up, "This is it. Do you want me to read it to you?" "Sure", I said in a bit of a stupor. In my mind I was waiting to hear what happened through this miraculous Fairy Tale I was living. Fairy Tale in that I was a miracle sitting upright, okay, supported upright, in this temporary berth. Fairy Tale because soon I was going to go home after being told just a few short days ago, I had less than "a 20% chance of making it off the table" and if I did make it through the surgery, I had an "80% chance of being in a vegetative state". I call this Miracle Fairy Tale Stuff for sure.

Pattie tenderly opened the envelope as if she had been handed a great secret held within be it the upcoming Oscar winner or maybe even the White House nuke code. Her graceful, steady fingers unfurled the trifold bleached white paper. She took another breath on top of the breath she was already holding and started reading. As she went on interpreting the foreign language both she and Doris obviously understood, tears started to flow. Doris meanwhile was laughing and smiling with spontaneous "Yeahs" here and there. They were the Yin and Yang of each other.

"I know what Dr. Kobrine said but I wasn't going to believe it until I read the Op Report and here it is! Genie, BeanHead, this is really good news. Okay..." She continued illuminating aloud. Every now and then I understood a word here and there. Then cognition kicked in when words were being used describing the actual opening of my skull, the instruments used, the placement of my body and my head. Suddenly cellular memory kicked in with accompanying soundtrack and anesthesia scents of the OR. The fairy tale was turning into a not so happy little bit of a scary horror story. "Pattie, Honey, I'm feeling kinda like I'm going to pass out. I don't think I can hear anymore right now and be okay." "Okay, okay, I'll just sit here and read it to myself, 'cause I have got to finish it to really know you're okay." She patted my left thigh. Next thing I remember is closing my eyes and sometime later opening my eyes to see Pattie sitting with her eyes closed in the chair beside my bed with the opened envelope beneath the handheld Operative Report in her lap and a great big smile upon her catnapping face. Doris was in the chair at the foot of my bed looking like a sleeping princess. All was right with the world. The Fairy Tale was true.

Pattie waited all day for a copy of that report so that she could believe in writing what she had been told in verse. Actually, knowing Pattie, she had been waiting since Dr. Arthur Kobrine, my mighty Neurosurgeon, stepped into the family waiting room four days earlier shortly after the completion of our 6 plus hours in surgery. She waited and waited some more to know I was going to be okay. She could have been home doing laundry, or out on a date, or hanging with Doris somewhere. Instead, she had spent her day off from the hospital in another hospital with me waiting to scrutinize what she had been told so she could believe in black and white what was before her eyes.

She loves me....

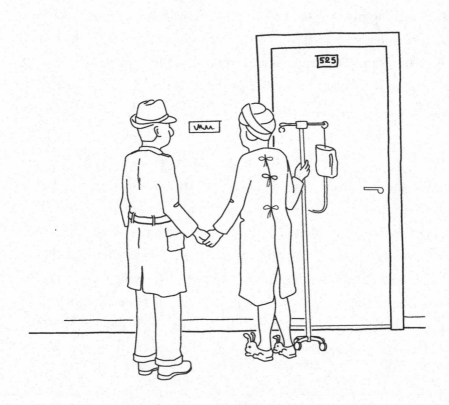

Don't tell me, he's dead now...

They're Dead Now

It was Tuesday, five days since my craniotomy, and I could not stop crying. Being in a complete fog as to why I was crying made wanting to cry all that much more necessary, it seemed. I sat crossed-legged, turban-headed, not knowing what I looked like in the middle of my hospital bed on the fifth floor, where brain tumor people go, in George Washington University Medical Hospital, Washington, DC.

"Why can't I stop crying? I am so happy to be alive. I am here. My heart is filled with gladness and I can't stop crying.", I asked pleading for an answer through the deluge and snot. Cassandra, (I worked very hard to remember every one of my nurses through this journey and to this day I still do), who had come into my room ready with vitals and meds, sat beside me on the bed. She was the first nurse who touched me, really touched me, outside the mandatory touch nurse zone since I had arrived last Wednesday evening. She wrapped her loving arms around me allowing me to rest my broken head on her shoulder and weep like a baby. "I don't know Honey, but you go ahead and cry it all out." Shortly after that it was time for her to go home as it was almost 7:00 am and her overnight shift was complete. She came back to check on me one more time before she left, gave me a kiss on my forehead, a squeeze on my hands and said in her beautiful Havana accent, "You're alright child. Don't worry."

It was about 11:00 am when Dr. Arthur Kobrine, my neurosurgeon, came in for his daily post-op visit. There I was still sitting in the middle of the bed, wailing like a running river. "What are you crying for?", he asked in a rather stern voice. "I don't know. I'm so happy and I can't stop crying." "Well, stop it!", he said with a loud jolt in his voice and a scowl across his face. Well, that was a shocker and I found it to be rather rude. "You can't talk to me that way! You can't yell at me! I just had brain surgery!"

One of the nurses, new to me that day, was standing behind him flashing a secret smile as if should he see it, she would be either tossed out the fifth-floor window or immediately fired. Dr. Kobrine suddenly turned, shoulders slightly hunched over, left the room abruptly without even looking over my chart or me.

About ten minutes later two more amused nurses came in the room asking, "What did you say to him?" When I told them, they totally cracked up in laughter. "Why?" "No one has ever spoken to him like that before. He came out of your room laughing so hard he had to lay his head down on the nurses station counter. We've never seen him laugh."

Late afternoon now and Dad walked in. He was stopping by to visit after his patient office hours and before heading home, so it was well after 5:00 pm. Dad, Dr. Alfred John Suraci, MD, was a magnificent reconstructive surgeon, an authentic Life Healer. Meanwhile, his daughter was a recent brain surgery survivor still sitting in the middle of her bed, unceasingly bawling. He sat cross legged in the chair up against the wall at the foot of my bed.

Coming in from the gray, snowy, dingy D.C. day Dad still had on his beige London Fog raincoat with the brown leather houndstooth buttons. All except for one that was a herringbone pattern, which he had so proudly replaced not Mom. As always upon his head, he was wearing his signature adorable dark brown fedora hat. Again, my stumbling snotty petition: "Dad, I can't stop crying. I have been crying all day. I don't want to cry. I have no reason to cry. I survived! I'm alive! I am so happy to be here, yet I can't stop crying. And it hurts. So, why can't I stop crying?" He had been leaning on the arm of the chair with his right arm and now his left hand was sneaking a move up to cover his mouth. "And you're laughing at me!" I said pointing my right index finger straight at him.

"Genie, Honey, this is normal. It's called post-operative depression and it's no big deal. Everybody gets it. It will pass soon." The flood gates instantly shut closed. "It's normal?" My shoulders dropped out of my ears, I could feel my neck come out of its turtle like shell, my tears immediately dried and I felt a brightness that I knew had embraced me from the moment I consciously woke from surgery, the Light of Bliss. "Okay." was my emphatic response. "Then walk me", I implored with a smile.

No one, NO ONE, in all the world has this walk with my Dad but me. He never combed or brushed my hair like he did my other three sisters. Actually, that's a good thing, 'cause it may just be possible he would never had been able to perform life healing surgery if he had tried being I am an Italian Botticelli Celtic waves curly girl, but I digress. He never took me to a Father-Daughter Breakfast, Dinner or Dance as he had the others. He never just sat with me cause that's all he wanted to do but right here, right now, my Dad was going to walk me, and it was just us. He helped me out of bed, arranging the IV's still connected in my arms along with the rolling transport pole. I slipped into my bunny slippers and we were off, real slow. Really, real slow. I held onto the IV pole with my right hand and Dad held onto me on my left.

There we were, not saying a word, as my Dad was always, shall we say, at a loss of words around me. We were strolling, as if sedated (one of us was), down the hall of the fifth floor Brain Department of the hospital he had worked in for years after graduating from George Washington University Medical School. The same hospital I was born in. As we approached a patient room on the right Dad obviously wanted to make his way over to read the plaque to the left of the door. He seemed pensive as he read, "Ah, that's Dr. (so and so 'cause I don't remember) and his wife. I knew them. They're dead now." "Oh, I'm sorry Dad." We continued to shuffle coming yet to another door on the right with a plaque to the left. I just knew he had to see it. "Uh, that's Dr. (so and so some more) and his wife. I knew them. They're dead now." "Oh, I'm sorry, Dad." At this point I'm thinking, this could be unpleasant should it continue. Well, here we were at door number three. Guess what? They're dead now too. Well, damn, this could get to be a real downer for Dad, seeing all his fellow classmates and lifelong medical comrades in his face plaque dead. Number four and I just can't even say it anymore, mostly cause I am about to crack up laughing but that certainly could be taken the wrong way. By door number five it just came out, "Don't tell me...They're dead now."

Together the twinkle in our eyes danced as we both totally burst out laughing. He'd been waiting for that knowing I was trying my best to be compassionate but hey, somewhere after door number four and right there at door number five compassion twisted into a very sick sense of humor that seems to be prevalent in medical families from time to time.

We made the U-turn at the end of the corridor heading back to Room 525 (kinda crazy knowing that was also my apartment number when I was living in New York City). As we slow-mo NASCAR-ed up the hallway the two of us were holding onto each other as we came upon each doorway with standard plaque to the left. No words necessary but laughter was getting to the point of having to be told to be quiet or we'll have to separate you two, as there were patients needing their rest.

Daddy helped me back into bed rearranging the IV pole, placing a pillow below my knees and bolstering several behind my back keeping me in a upright position so as to prevent any brain seepage. As he covered me with blankets, he kissed my checks, both sides of course being of Italian descent, turned and left for the night.

I watched as his small body walked away. A new and very special Daddy-Daughter Love swelled up inside me that had never existed before. I knew all in one full sweep I had just experienced my Daddy combing and brushing my hair, my longed-for Father-Daughter Dinner Dance and a love for this daughter unlike any love he had ever felt before in his life.

I have that Daddy Walk Me Moment. Nobody else has that. So when my other sisters talk about their times with our Dad, I no longer have that left out but I'm okay feeling. Instead deep inside my soul I smile a really big all-embracing heart smile because I am the only one who has this ultimately unique slow split second in life, Dad and Me Moment. I treasure my, "Genie, Honey, that's normal, Walk me, They're dead now" stroll with my Dad.

Baseball Head

Give them a job. Give everybody I love and who loves me a job. That's what I thought. My premise was, should I die, which having been told I had "less than a 20% chance of making off the table", it would keep them busy versus sitting around the funeral parlor lamenting, "This sucks. She died." And, if through surviving surgery I slipped into a vegetative state, which I had been told I had an 80% chance of doing, again it would keep them occupied and again they would not be sitting around presuming, "This really sucks! She's a veg." What really sucked about that scenario is I would more than likely hear them from this side of life in my own new world, saying, "This sucks" about me. Oh no you don't! Give them a job. And if I should be blessed as our prayers raised up to survive my brain surgery being given a chance to create a new fully functioning life, different yet functioning, I will need help through recovery. So, giving them jobs is super important because I want them to love their temporary per diem position so much they won't be thinking, "This job sucks! When is she going to be okay again so I can stop doing this?"

Way back when Kenny and I were early dating he taught me a lesson that was bigger than I could take in at first, yet had I not studied it, processed it and made it my own to a elevated degree, I never would have survived my brain surgery. The lesson: "Until you learn to receive equal to what you give, you are not truly giving". Equal exchange, how's that smack ya'?

As I approached the day of my surgery, looking from all sides, I could imagine all possibilities and scenarios. Putting myself in their place, I wanted to believe my gift to those lovingly involved was my letting go allowing them to care for me.

My fellow fashionista sister, Terry, accepted the job of taking care of my hair. We had no idea what my hair or head was going to look like once the turban was removed. Plan A: Doctor Kobrine would shave the right side of my head leaving an inch or two strips of hair in front of the ear so that we could do the bald man comb over with the long hair on the left side of my head. Our thought was no one would ever be able to tell I was half bald. Silly us. Picture this, my hair was nearly waist length cut in a half moon trim prior to the shave.

Early morning of the sixth day after my craniotomy one of Dr. Kobrine's interns cut my turban off. I will never forget the moment, his face, the scissors, the sounds, my head's tenderness and my emotional feelings. Terry showed up right on time for work that afternoon with comb, brush and trimming scissors in hand. That's brave, fashionista and fearless. I'm not looking at it and it's not like she's seen it before, but you would have thought from her approach that she'd seen it a hundred times and knew exactly what to do, no problem. She climbed up onto my hospital bed getting a good seating behind me. I had no idea what my head or any hair looked like. Nor was I ready to know. I was just seated pretty and happy to be alive. Terry started doing whatever it was she was doing. Now and again I heard a clip here, a clip of hair there. She was talking her, 'I'm just fine' way of talking when she is a little outside her usual life stream and I thought, *Well, that's normal, so can't be too bad.*

Every now and then, there was a tug which I am sure I would never have noticed had my head not been so sensitive, but it was, so each tug was followed by a spontaneous low tone slight gasp. Each tiny quick inhale prompted a litany of "I'm sorry Honey, I'm so sorry." "No worry", as I patted her thighs. My hands were resting on her to steady myself and for the needed reassurance that all was well. Terry was doing her being in charge of my hair job better than anyone else in all the world and I knew that. Certainly better than I could do.

At one point after a long silence between us, as she was lifting and shifting what hair was there ever so gently, she said; "Ya know, it's really not all that bad... You just look like a baseball from behind." We both in a flash of a moment straightened up as we held our breath wondering from both sides now, 'Is it okay, to say something like that?' Flash over, we totally cracked up in laughter holding tightly to each other's hands. I was so happy, and I felt so fully secure and loved while Terry was taking such good care of me, my hair and my head.

A good six months later Terry told me, "I wasn't about to tell you right then and there, but tangles and wads of your hair were coming out in my hands as it was obviously just all matted up cut and uncut under the turban. I didn't want to freak you out, so I stuffed it into my jean pockets while sitting behind you." When she told me that I totally broke out in laughter. The very thought of her stuffing gross, bloody hair into her jean pockets probably not remembering until she got home taking her jeans off getting ready for bed that night was quite the vision. Total gross out! Fashionista, brave and compassionate. Meanwhile I was absolutely okay in my thought process if I were totally bald for the rest of my life and we just needed to shine up my head every now and then. Who cares if I have hair? I'm alive! I'm alive and not a vegetable. I'm alive, not a vegetable, recovering well after major brain surgery and I have a baseball head to prove it.

Thanksgiving Eve
Going Home Kinda

I remember waking to them standing around my bed. Not a dream, reality. "So many men. So little time." I actually said that out loud to the eight interns, residents, aka Dr. Arthur Kobrine's baby doctors surrounding my bedside the morning of possible discharge from G. W. University Medical Center. *I'm a much funnier girl since brain surgery,* I heard myself think. *What part of my brain got tickled for that to happen?* The boys laughed while they proceeded to touch my head oooing and ahhhing. I couldn't help wondering if they were the same folks who had been in the surgical arena early morning six days ago yet could not form thought to word fast enough to ask. One remarked how clean a cut it was and how tight the skull laid back in tack. "That's the Kobrine trademark", another said. *He's either teacher's pet or a suck-up,* I chuckled to myself. "It really is beautiful", the headcheese (pun intended) of rounds said twinkling a smile in my direction. "Everything is looking so good. Time for you to go home." "I can call Kenny to come get me?" "Make the call."

1989 was of course before we started carrying our tiny, little phones with us everywhere we went. It is not clear in my memory how I made the call just that I made the call. "Hi Honey, guess what? I can leave today. Now!" We both smiled big through the handheld, attached to the wall by wires phones. "Give me a little bit of time while I get everything ready and I'm on my way." We made our conversation brief so as to cause no delay, yet I do remember saying; "Get me out of here or I'm gonna die." To which Kenny replied; "Put your best, I'm all better on and I'm coming to get you." This is Kenny's favorite split-second moment through the brain surgery experience.

It seemed I was sitting and waiting, sitting and waiting, sitting and waiting, rocking in the middle of my bed forever and a day. Where is he? I was lingering with halted breath, spying the portal entrance, listening for his footsteps to walk in the door prepared to whisk me away from literally all the bone-chilling, hair-raising events into the new narrative of our life. It was hours since my call. Where is he? My anxiety was leveling up with thoughts of he may not be coming at all today, maybe not until tomorrow or later. Then it might be too late.

Finally, he sashayed in looking ever so fine in jeans and his denim jacket. Crowning his dark, thick hair was the very black leather tam he wore the first day we spotted each other August 31, 1977, in the halls of Anne Arundel Community College. "*O'loui!*", I sighed. "Looking good!" Meanwhile I was wearing my blue silk-like grown up lingerie, a what was called then hot pink tie at the waist robe and my now infamous bunny slippers. The man took a little longer than expected so that "everything would be perfect" for my departure, my arrival and so he would look his best as my loving chaperone homeward. I barely recall the wheelchair ride but what I do remember most intensely was the first whiff of fresh air. Oh My! Fresh, real, chill on the face and cold to the hands, up the nose fresh air!

We traveled through DC to my parent's Maryland home. Staying with them was Dad's idea approved by Mom. I needed 24/7 around the clock watch which meant both Kenny and I had to shut down our businesses. When Dad heard that was our beginning plan for the first few weeks, his response was, "Well that's kind of stupid. Why don't you come stay with your Mom and me?" Dad was a Doctor and Mom a Nurse. They knew I would get much better intimate care from them than in the hospital as wonderful as infirmary personnel was. They also knew something was happening recovery wise, but neither could they diagnose just what, just yet. Thus, I was allowed to leave within the week versus the original two week proposed stay. "Kenny and Beau, (our magnificent Bearded Collie puppy dog), can come stay every night after work." Such a generous gifting from big, generous hearts.

What I remember of the first real fresh air car ride was just how in tune I was with our Beau who loved hanging his head out the passenger side window. I was doing the same to catch every bit of good time reality in the outside world I could feel through every sense, five and more, my heart beating happy dance as never before. So it was through our Nation's Capital streets passing right by the White House residence on 16th and Constitution, this half bald, scar headed woman, looking a bit like a character from the Rocky Horror show, in the hot pink bath robe with bunny slippers was hanging out the car window, big ol' tongue exposed trying to catch the snowflakes as they tasseled to the ground.

I'm not sure how long my Mom had been waiting on the front steps. Possibly as long as her last conversation with Kenny about our leave and feasible ETA. I can still hear my Mother's gasp upon our arrival as she saw my exposed bald head perched out the passenger side window. When she caught a glimpse of my less than snowy winter attire, she ran back inside to grab a blanket wrapping it around me as she and Kenny assisted my walk up the steps of the front porch. "Honey, it's cold out here! Let's get you inside!"

Oh! What a Heavenly Thanksgiving Eve going home kinda, ride it was!

Little Stories — Big Memories
Hospital Short Stories

I Could Have Jumped a Plane?

My poor Mom was frantic. Ken and I were 45 minutes "late" getting to George Washington University Hospital Center for my admission Wednesday evening, the night before my craniotomy. We were to be there by 6:00 pm. We walked in the front door at 6:45pm. "Where have you been? I thought for sure you climbed onto a plane and flew away!" *Wow! Seriously? Why would you think that of me? There's an idea I never had, although it's not a bad one.* "Honey, you have to be here, you have no choice!" Big clue for succeeding in life. Don't ever tell a Leo, especially a double Leo, they have no choice. I remember the glare my Lioness personality, shall we say, glistened in that moment. "Oh yes I do have a choice.", my mane ruffling. "I most assuredly have the choice of not being here right now. I chose to be here right now even though I don't want to be. So do not tell me I have no choice. I do." On a good day we were an hour and a half away farm to city. We were late due to the really big snowstorm blanketing Washington, D.C. In afterthought glancing at my Mother's frightened face, my protectress Leo Lioness Mom, trying to soften the blow, I queried, "I could have gotten on a plane and flown away?" Although had I known the plane thing was a possibility would I have hopped that plane? No, I made the right choice. Always remember you do have a choice. Be brave in your choosing. You are powerful.

I Crazy Love It!

For six plus hours I'm under anesthesia having a craniotomy, brain surgery. To amuse themselves my husband, Kenny, and my baby sister, Pattie, who have a crazy wonderful relationship since day one of meeting each other, amused themselves with coming up with a new nickname for me. Six hours mind you and my new nick name is... BeanHead...Beaners for short. They love me. And I crazy love it!

Whole Body Smile

I remember the first day, that I remember, Dr. Arthur Kobrine coming in to see me post-surgery during his rounds. It was Sunday after my surgery on Thursday. That is not to say that was his first post-surgical visit. It is the first one I remember. There he stood all tall, lanky and stiff as a board at the foot of my hospital bed. There I was balancing on all four crawling on top of the covers toward him, turban head and IV in tow. That in and of itself could have freaked him out. I arrived at my destination, pulled up onto my knees and put my arms around his waist giving a big ol' hug of gratitude. His long arms just hung by his side. The man did not know what to do with that. "And then you do this", I said, as I picked up his arms at his wrist placing them behind my back completing the full circle of hug. The nurse in attendance took a step back like maybe he was going to implode or something. What I remember most in that moment is feeling his whole-body smile.

The Healing Yin and Yang of Hand Holding

Ahh, Sunday afternoon I remember waking from time to time through hours of peaceful sleep feeling my turbaned head on the upright pillow.

Kenny was holding my hand on the left of me and Terry holding my hand on the right of me. For hours neither let go. I would wake and there they would be like bookends on your favorite library shelf supporting your best-loved, first choice reads. One time I would wake and they were talking low and soft. Another time, in silence, they were watching TV. Yet another and they would be carrying on laughing about something. Once in a while, they and the room were in total serene quietude. Each time neither let go of my hands. Total deep, abiding, comfort, love and joy. The Healing Yin and Yang of Hand Holding.

The Brick Wall Hits Back

The view from my hospital room window to the left of where I sat supported in bed was a brick wall. It is actually quite amazing what you can learn about the outside world from looking at a brick wall. The changing shading shapes from the sun upon the stockade tell of the time of day. The shadows from the evening lights spin silhouettes good for making up stories in the middle of the night. I made friends with that brick wall. Admittedly there were times my emotions hit her ruddy crimson bulkhead. Sometimes she threw them right back at me. I suppose I wasn't the first. It may not be easy being a brick wall outside a hospital room window.

Slippers & Sis

Folks loved my bunny slippers. I loved my bunny slippers. I bought them with me because they reminded me of little Slippers, the baby bunny sister of big Sis, the angora bunny girls Kenny gave me for our seventh Wedding Anniversary waiting for me back home. You know, number seven is wool. As I rehearsed walking, holding onto my IV pole down the hall and back of the fifth floor Brain Ward, folks would shout out from their sequestered rooms, "Love your slippers!" Amazing how pure, simple love can fill one's feels good cup.

I Will Haunt You

Possibly it was Monday, maybe Tuesday, after brain surgery last Thursday. A nurse or nurse attendant, who I had never seen before nor after, came in "encouraging" me to get up out of bed to go to the bathroom. No problem, I thought, as I had done pretty good with assistance standing on my own. So, I slipped into Slippers and Sis as we shuffled into the little white room with the thin hanging threads for pulling when in need of assistance. She then backed out and closed the door. "Hello. Where did you go?" "I'm right out here, outside the door." I knew that and was highly uncomfortable with it. "Hello. Just had brain surgery. Lots of porcelain in here. Would appreciate your help." "No, you go ahead. I'm right outside the door." *Seriously! Brain surgery! Still unsteady! Connected to IV pole! Where is your compassion?* "I would really appreciate your help in here." "No, you go ahead. I'm right outside the door." She was obviously uncomfortable with seeing a human being's bare ass and I was pissed. "OK, I tell you what. If I fall, hit my head and die in here after surviving brain surgery, I will come back and haunt you." "OK, I'm right outside the door." At least I will know where to find her, right outside the door.

Chapter Three

After Brain Surgery (ABS)
Me And My Brain Living The Good Life
Most of the Time

Thanksgiving Day Tub Time

There I was sitting butt-naked in Mom and Dad's master bathtub with both my Husband and Mother bathing me, mid-morning Thanksgiving Day. Mom's goal was to teach Kenny how to take care of my head. To that, she and Kenny had lent a helping hand getting me up out of bed and climbing the twenty-four steps up the winding staircase to Mom and Dad's second floor bedroom.

Oh Dear God! Water, warm, body wrapping water. Sigh... Ever so carefully with their assistance I was eased down into the pure pleasure of soaking luxury caressing every cell of my being. I listened, more like heard, the heart tender motherly nurse-like instructions as Mom gently touched my head. I could tell by the slight tinges of tenderness my blessed skull may be a bit sore for a while. "You have to be so careful, Ken, when cleaning her head, so take this washcloth and..." She continued stroking my head with the thermal towel. Have you ever felt a warm, slightly wet towel lay upon your bald head? It is Heavenly. Sitting there, I felt like a baby in their first tub atop a kitchen counter, well, until I looked down upon my adult woman body in view. Babies don't have hair down there nor boobie girls up there. I took a cavernous breath in and out thinking to myself, *Well, here's a place I never imagined being, butt naked in my parent's tub with both my mother and husband in the same room with me.*

Meanwhile as I sat upright bits of blood and messy whatever stuff dropped off into the water encircling me. That was kinda gross, so I thought, *Look over there. Look anywhere but into the water right now.* I gazed up at my Mom and Kenny above me. Their four kind hands touching and caring for my head in unison, two the teacher, two the student. Mine and my Mom's eyes met. I remember the wrinkles of concern on her forehead and the sadness in her eyes. I can only imagine how a Mother would feel with her grown daughter sitting in her tub seemingly unable to bathe herself, looking as I did with a half bald darned stitched head. My husband may have been thinking, 'This could be the way it is for a good long while or maybe even the rest of our life.' Not so, yet for now, for me, this was Nirvana.

Their voices fell quiet. Mom leaned over the tub with a soft pink hand towel whispering close to my ear, "Here Honey, this is for your privacy." *Say what? I'm butt naked literally, bald head to toes, with both my mother and my husband in the same bathroom serenely bathing me and what?* Arms raised waist high, I received the mini-cloth with both outstretched hands as my eyes met the compassionate giver. The smile that blossomed across my face and the laughter in my eyes questioned her in silence, *What do I do with this? What parts of my birthday suit is this teensy weeny chamois to conceal? Why shroud at this point in the process? What privacy?* As she read my mind the sheer delight of her empathy through the ridiculousness of action set in.

She turned laughing so freely she had to grab the door frame to remain upright as she retreated from the room leaving Kenny and myself to the task at hand and head.

Forever I will remember Kenny's gentle touch lifting me from the basin as if I may break, allowing me to lean into him while he towel dried my energy-weakened body. My mind was blank as to how I got into the bed with fresh pajamas. What I did know was I had been deeply cared for by two of the most loving people in my life and now it was time for me to close my eyes and sleep on this consecrated morning of giving thanks.

Hours later muffled sounds of talk and laughter whispered through the bedroom door. There was a holiday celebration taking place on the other side. I was content to remain right where I was nestled in soft, clean, fresh scented bed linens versus the stiff bleached hospital starched sheets. I laid in a cozy room sleepy eyed gazing at the grand artist Fall explosion of color outside the front window of the guest room in my parent's home. Oops, there I go again, slipping into the fog of waking gone, ahhh.

Now and again taking a break from the feast before them, someone would peak their head in the room checking in on me. Dad, Pattie, Terry, Richard, Michael, Brendan, Erin, and more times than anyone else Mom and Kenny. Eyes closed, my ears slightly attuned yet wearily being so close to the brain, I heard Aunt Lilly, "Honey, you've got to eat. Wake up. You've got to eat something."

The following day there were stories full of laughter about how Aunt Lilly tried to force feed me, afraid I may die right in front of her if I didn't partake in the full out throttle holiday feast. The last thing my body wanted was food. Sleep, real sleep was high on my to-do list. So, it was I continued to slip in and out of intense daytime napping mode. Kenny did bring a plate to my bedside, a lovely palate of color, basking in a multitude of invitational aromas, my Mother's lovingly created festival nourishment. Yet as he raised a fork to my mouth within a moment of waking, I was gone again traveling to la-la land. The prescribed take home heavy drugs were kicking in. I was exhausted beyond my own knowing and my body surrendered into its needs. The day of smiling fog done. The family crowd dispersed to their own home abodes. The night dark, Kenny came in and laid beside me in the twin bed, his left arm across my body, head upon my shoulder. He gave me a kiss upon my cheek. I smiled and was gone again being gently swallowed by the very essence of gratitude for my first Thanksgiving Day after the beginning of my new life on earth.

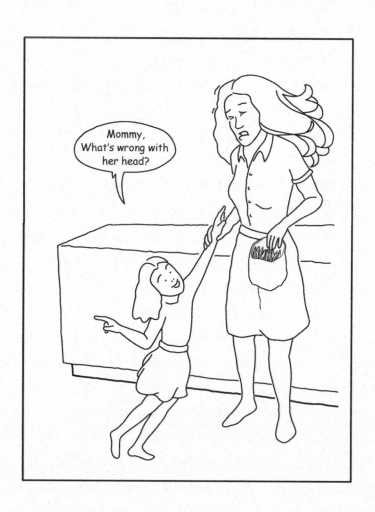

Mommy, What's Wrong With Her Head?

Testing...Testing...Time for another Test of How Ya' Simply Doin'?

It was a slow day in Davidsonville, Maryland so we decided to take a little elementary test time out into the world. We drove to Basics, our grocery store in Crofton, for a trial run of sending me in with a daily breads list and a certain amount of money. The passing grade would be if I were to come back out with the correct inventory of items on the checklist and the accurate amount of capital, hard, cold cash in hand.

Meanwhile, Kenny could keep an eye on me through the front full glass wall from The Husband Lane as we called it. Anyone else calls it the yellow lined Fire Lane, the one in front of most retail establishments, but we knew well I wasn't going in for Fire.

So, one last look into Kenny's eyes before opening the passenger side door, and off I went on my own, brave, courageous and a true believer that I could at least accomplish goal Number 1, the Food List. If it reads beans get beans not radishes. Big inhale, pulling the door open. Hey, it was a country store at the time. No magical I see you coming automated doorways, although we were the first to bring your own, as long as it has the Basics Logo on it, cloth grocery bags.

Once inside I looked over the 4-item list as if studying for the SAT. Number 1, Green Beans... Scan produce on the left...I see'm! I think. I am halfway there at least on #1. The words "green beans" on paper...Brain file search for green beans...Got it...Scrutinize...Scan... Locate...Get there...Retrieve. Green Beans in real 3D form. The sign says so right above them. Must be. I am walking to the green beans.

As I approach, I notice a woman and a young child with just about a full bag of beans. Okay, no invading space. No grabbing. Sashaying toward my first prize I was remembering (I was remembering!) what Kenny's Mom said one day when we went grocery shopping together. She watched me purposefully pick the beans versus just grab-bagging.

With a smirk upon her face Mother proudly stated, "Well, I certainly do know that Kenny eats the best green beans available." Why get less? Why give less? I was feeling ever so pleased with myself picking the best beans and placing them in the little brown Basics bag made just for such a purpose when suddenly I noticed out of the corner of my eye because I can, because I now have peripheral vision, that the woman with the almost full bag has laid it down beside the bay of beans and is leaving the produce area rather stealthily. She is also under her breath with a tone of angst, fear, and a demanding tight lip frustration, whispering to her daughter, "Get over here. Get over here right now!"

I had decided earlier in the day to give my head a hat rest, so yes, my half bald, Mrs. Frankenstein stitched skull was exposed to the world. The little girl of 3 or 4 was just standing there in all her glory, staring at my head asking, "Mommy, what's wrong with her head?" Mommy meanwhile was kinda Two-Fold freaking out. One-Fold, Holy Crap! She touched the same bay o'beans I'd been picking from and Two-Fold, my child is not allowing me to sneak away from the grotesqueness of it all. I on the other hand was having my own Two-Fold thought process. One-Fold, I just wanted to run after that woman with my head, front and center, saying, "You can't catch a brain tumor!" and Two-Fold, your child asked a question, just answer it.

As much as I really wanted to One-Fold it, I was cool and instead jumped right into Two-Fold answering this adorable, honest, no bones about it little girl's inquiry. "I had a boo-boo in my head and the doctor took care of it and I am all better now." I smiled down at her and she beamed with her new knowledge right back up at me. We had a moment of soul connection right there in front of the green bean sanctuary. "Oh" she twinkled in an upward tone of sweetness and skipped off to meet up with her still under tone, commanding, freaking, should know better at your age but you don't, mom. I smiled in her direction but as soon as her little girl was close enough, mom grabbed her hand and whisked her around the corner into the cereal aisle as the little girl waved good-bye and blew a kiss of Thank You in my direction. Having never experienced a brain tumor craniotomy survivor in the produce section before, mom probably did a similar freak out when she saw the Frankenberry cereal box on the shelf next to the Fruit Loops in her escape corridor.

I do not remember #2, 3 nor 4 on my pilot trial grocery list. All that mattered in the moment was the purity of that little girl's soul riding deep within my heart. She asked a question, a basic, in her mind essential, open, honest question right there in Basics bean basin section of life. And I got to answer her vital, fundamentally important query on her enthusiastic level of understanding. That's all she needed. She had no 'I have been living long enough to be an adult' judgement nor fear. Her only concern in all the world was, there's something I do not know. Tell me and I will listen. Thank you and done, moving on, gotta go. The pure heart of a child.

Shortly thereafter I made it to the register where the cashier was sweet, tender and patient with me in regard to the money counting, as were the folks standing in line behind me. She took the time to show me between paper receipt and money in hand I did it right. After that day in sheer gratitude I always made the intentional attempt to go to her line when cashing out.

As I left the store walking to the car still parked in The Husband Lane, (who knows how long I had been in there?) I could see Kenny smiling through the passenger side window. When I saw the expression upon his face the one word that immediately came forward on the blackboard in my mind written in big, bold letters was "Relief". I know we said the Test that day was about the grocery list and the correct change, but I could tell he was thinking seizure. Big exhale of happiness, as he thought, "With all the activity in there, she did not seizure." Test day for Kenny too.

So it was that day and many days forward Kenny sat in The Husband Lane with a Two-Fold purpose: One-Fold, watch her every move for safety and concern and Two-Fold, can't wait to hear the story she comes out with this time. Hearing just the basics in The Husband Lane, where else, other than at Basics.

Fireworks In My Brain

To this day I am only halfway excited about fireworks. I love the brilliant colors and the expanding upward swirl of the trajectory but the other half, the roaring boom and swirling sound of the aftermath is a heart pounding cellular memory I cannot explain to anyone when they experience my potent fear in its presence. As a child, our parents faithfully made the yearly trek to the Washington Monument Grounds with all seven kids for the Fourth of July extravaganza. While I marveled in awe at the sight of such vibrant pizzazz blasting through the night sky, I was also the child standing on the Army blanket locked kneed, body shaking on the Potomac Tidal Basin Grounds wailing uncontrollably, tiny hands over my ears screaming into the rather startled crowd, "Stop it! Stop it! It's like war! Make it stop!" Once again giving not only my parents but six other siblings reason for not claiming me as one of their own clan. Where that came from to be propelled out from the mouth of a single digit aged child can only be attributed to an earlier recollection. What did I know of war at such a tender age in the early 1950's, Washington, DC?

Fast forward roughly 4 decades. Kenny and I are party positioned on the brownstone rooftop of a friend's townhouse in Baltimore, Maryland just as the Fourth of July Fireworks commence over the Harbor. As we were far enough away from ground zero, sounds were dulled to the point of my total enjoyment of sight low sound. Admittedly I could barely contain my excitement! As seeing not hearing I finally had something to compare and explain to others what happened on a daily basis inside my head. "Kenny! Kenny! That's it! That's what I am living inside my head! That's what I see from inside!" I was totally thrilled finally being able to describe what I had tried for so long to explain in theory. Kenny on the other hand, well, his face said it all even before he spoke, "That's Not Okay! You have to go see Kobrine this week and tell him. That can't be good!" While I throughly appreciated his loving concern, I on the other hand, loved it. Without the excruciating sounds of annihilation, I considered it a wondrous world of awe-inspiring contemplative sparkles, commonsensical fairies and pure pleasure.

At this point in time we were nearly five years post craniotomy. I was doing quite well as far as I was concerned yet everytime I articulated this thought of fireworks in my brain to Kenny, he did not share my enthusiasm. There were times we would be talking, and a thought would cross my mind that seemed appropriate to introduce and Voila! Sparks! Pyrotechnics! culminating in big happy eyes and a ginormous smile. Sometimes the conversation continued along its projected path. Other times it took a left turn into 'I haven't a clue as to what I was going to say' alley ways. Just in case, I made the appointment, drove into DC and spoke with my tall, thin, lanky-armed, sure-handed neurosurgeon, Dr. Arthur Kobrine. "Okay, I'm sure you have heard this before, but Kenny said we need to check this out with you 'cause he doesn't think it sounds good. When I have a thought, I get fireworks in my brain. It's like a spark sets off. The colors are fabulous, breathtaking, absolutely mind-blowing! Sometimes who knows what thought I was having because sometimes I remember it and sometimes I am oblivious as to where I was going with whatever started it all."

The good doc leaned back as he often did when about to strike his, 'I'm thinking' pose. He folded his long extended left arm over his solar plexus, placed his right hand up to his chin with eyes slightly closed as if squinting made his mind think more clearly. Clarity did come through, after a momentary undertone of hum. "That's perfect! I have never heard it expressed that way, but it makes perfect sense." *What is it that is making perfect sense*, I thought, as I observed the glitter of brilliance in my brain before I had the chance to mouth the words. "That makes perfect sense" he said again. "When I cut into your brain to remove the tumor, of course I had to slice through blood vessels, arteries, and synapses. When that occurs, the straightforward thought process is interrupted. The moment of fireworks you are experiencing, and that is a perfect way of expressing it, is the thought jumping from one nerve ending to the other, like across the abyss, to continue the thought. The snap, the spark, the fireworks are in between the jump, the leap of the thought leaving one side and before its completion on the other side. Usually thought just flows because there is a continuous pathway to do so but after brain surgery those pathways have been disturbed. Your brain will rebuild new roads but until then, the thought has to take the leap of faith from one side of synapses to the other." Voila! Fireworks In My Brain! "Can I keep them?" I asked with a childlike desire already knowing the adult answer. I wanted to keep them forever. Keeping them forever, would always remind me what a grand and wondrous thing the mind inside my brain is. It makes fireworks all by itself without me...Well, wait...I was going to say, without me even thinking about it but, it's because I am thinking that it designs, generates, and gives birth to the fireworks. Awesome!

The fireworks in my brain eventually faded, no matter how much wishing I did that they wouldn't. Nowadays, when I expose myself by choice to Fourth of July Fireworks or anytime to celebrate fireworks, as they seem to have become quite popular throughout the calendar year, as long as I am far enough away from the deafening boom, be it outside or on TV with mute employed, I remember the delight of thought we simply don't even think about, the magic of making thought in and of itself. Meditate long enough on that and believe me fireworks of gratitude will explode in your brain.

One Zero One Zero
1010

The day was quiet and calm as I sat in Kenny's office working the books. Adding numbers as I had been for three years, now seven since my craniotomy, I saw the "1" on the page and took it over to the calculator. I saw another number and moved it as well to the calculator. It was the best I could do to remember one number at a time for the distance between page and calculator no matter if the two were sitting in each other's laps. I was okay with that because I could do that. I knew that when I got all the numbers showing on that one line moved over to and entered into the calculator I could then hit the "+" sign and start again with another line of numbers and eventually all the additions and subtractions would be complete creating a Total. Sitting alone in serene silence I was feeling pretty good about this achievement when suddenly I realized without warning, fanfare nor horns a'tooting I had seen the number 1010, remembered it in its totality all the way over to the calculator pressing each number with separate fingers as if a pro and viewing its entirety right before my eyes. A welling of grand accomplishment pyrotechnics flared up and out of my body. I did 1010! One-Zero-One-Zero! I did that! I remembered all the way from the page to the calculator 4, four whole numbers without looking back to the page!

My inner senses went aflutter with what the brain reads, hears, sees, knows. What the mind interprets, the picture the brain takes like a camera versus what the mind recognizes on the inner chalk board behind my forehead. What the brain perceives versus what the mind understands. How they both hear. Total exhilaration consumed my very Being.

I grabbed the cordless phone laying on its receiver in the upper right hand corner of the desk. In an instant my fingers were on Speed Dial #1 for Kenny. Ahh, Speed Dial! It's great 'cause you do not have to remember anything like numbers. It's not so great 'cause you don't have to remember anything like numbers. "Kenny! Honey, I just did 1010!" He was pleased enough to be very excited for me and in truth for himself as he had supported my 1-0-1-0 for seven years. I knew to call Kenny first, number 1 because, he is my Number 1 and I wanted to. He is my Best Boyfriend, Lover, Husband, my 24/7 Support Angel, my very Best Buddy Ever and I knew my next call, my Number Two, would be an extended chatter conclave.

My #2 Speed Dial was Beamer, aka, Patricia Beamer O'Sullivan, aka, the freaky, bald woman in Dr. Kobrine's office the day of our first consult, my Brain Buddy Bookend. We were each other's Brain Buddy Bookends because her brain tumor was left frontal and mine was right temporal, occipital, parietal. We figured if we got our heads together we could keep all the knowledge and wisdom of the world in there as she would support the one side and I the other. We were the perfect collaboration cooperative partnership. When Beamer answered the phone I could hardly contain myself. "Beam, I just did 1010! One-Zero-One-Zero!" "Awesome! Wow! I did that last week!" The tête-à-tête went from there and if anyone other than ourselves were listening, they would have thought we were talking a alien language but we knew and totally understood between right and left hemisphere, bookend to bookend, what 1010, One-Zero-One-Zero was really all about!

The Tumor Is Gone

"What?"

"It's gone! I am not kidding you. The tumor is gone!"

From inside the MRI (Meditation Room Insolation) capsule I heard Tom's voice, "The tumor is gone." I opened my visionary eyes searching for Tom's image in the mirror poised above my head on the module ceiling angled just right to be able to see into Tom's Tech Room at Anne Arundel General Hospital, Annapolis Maryland. By the third time he said it I was also reading his lips. "I'm not kidding you. The tumor is gone. It's truly gone!"

This was Spring 1996, seven years post craniotomy. A silence fell between us. I was still watching Tom. His eyes were filled with excitement. He had yet to exhale as he continued to work his high-tech wizardry. The smile beaming across his face could float three dozen helium balloons and the laugh lines surrounding his eyes gave the Angels reason to sing.

I too had yet to exhale. Being that one must lay extremely still during the MRI (Mystical Radical Idea) process I thought the tears flowing down my cheeks may be enough movement to curtail our purpose, so total blow out happy dance melt down was out of the question. As it was, the light fantastic thoughts prancing in my head just may change all images created from this moment on. *Thank You, Father-Mother God. Seriously Wow! The biggest difference is Reiki, I can't wait to tell Kenny! Thank You! Thank You! Thank You!* Still in the background of my inward verbal sojourns, I could hear Tom, telecommunication mike on, "Wow! Wow, Wow, Wow! How does this happen? I've never seen this! Gone! Just gone!"

There had been a tendril of tumor left behind on my carotid artery as to take it would have been more dangerous with possible compromising negative consequences than leaving it. Over the years of MRI's (Magical Radiating Impressions) Our Team, including me,

Kenny, Tom, Vikki, Lauren (My 3 MRI - Magical Remarkable Illuminati) and of course Dr. Arthur Kobrine, my Neurosurgeon Genius, watched for any changes, growth, etc. of this little bugger making sure to keep the rest of my brain safe from harm.

Change did happen. Happy change happened!

As my MRI (Mirror Rep Idolizer) with contrast was complete, Tom practically skipped into the "You're On Your Own Room" sliding me out like a cabinet drawer. "I am not kidding you. It's gone.", he said this time with a quiet still reverence, eyes beaming.

My single thought was, *It had to be the Reiki. God-Stuff. Nothing else has been done. Nothing else has changed. Intention and Reiki.* Intention, Reiki, God-Stuff changes everything.

Kenny as always was faithfully waiting in the reception area engaging Lauren in some small talk, some up close and personal and always when appropriate "pun-ish-ment" jokes. Tom, Vikki and I walked out from the background together with my library of hard copy film under my arms. Tom said it first, "Kenny, it's gone." He smiled, turned and walked back through the double doors from whence we came repeating the words while shaking his head, "It's gone!"

"Kenny, it's gone, really gone!" I am not sure how long we held each other wrapped in the realm of soulful consummation. At last the long-held exhale had begun to polish itself off from years of fears. We quietly turned holding hands, walking side by side in near sunset to our car as if we had been reassured life was ours to continue boldly, bravely and possibly even this time undaunted. Our heads were swimming in our own soup of contentment.

The tumor was gone, truly gone!

Tumors, Babies, and Me

For years I had wanted to go to the American Brain Tumor Association (ABTA) Annual Conference for patients, professionals and caregivers. For years I didn't think I could manage it on my own as I am not one for crowds, noise, or large bright lights, nor writing fast in terms of taking notes for what I might learn and do not want to forget. But there I was, they had come to the Washington, DC area close to home. I had no travel excuse.

As I descended the hotel escalator looking into the crowd below contemplating, *What was I thinking*, a beautiful, fashion chic woman glanced up. She moved like silk over to the bottom of the mechanically sloping stairway watching my downhill glide. She waited having yet to take her eyes from the point at which they had met mine. Her smile radiated comfort from deep within her heart. As my feet met the stationary floor, she took my hand sliding me to the right out of the way of others making their descent. Perhaps from all the way up on the first floor prior to my nosedive into the Conference she felt my heart beating with anxiety of being alone in a crowd.

"I am so glad you came this year. Thank you." "Thank you for your efforts so that we might all be here to hear, listen and learn." While my outer voice replied rather sheepishly still trying to figure out why she chose me to zero in on, my inner voice asked, *Did I just use two different here/hears in the same sentence?* "My name is Naomi Berkowitz. I am the current President of ABTA." *Wow!*

Why had I hesitated all these years? Already there is sweet serenity and all I did was arrive in the room. So, with Naomi's help I looked over the program and highlighted those lectures of interest. I do not remember the exact title but the two words most prevalent in my wellness journey at the time were "Tumor" and "Baby". I know the word "Fertility" was in there somewhere. I thought, *Well, neither my neurosurgeon nor our reproductive endocrinologist knew anything to tell me, so maybe I will learn something for us to know through our pilgrimage moving forward.* My neurosurgeon had told us both pre- and post-craniotomy, "Had your baby lived and you continued the pregnancy while the tumor was still in you, both you and the baby would have died as the hormonal changes through your pregnancy would accelerate the tumors growth by 60% making it totally inoperable. Neither of you would have survived."

Never would I have imagined as I sat in a small packed room amidst hundreds of new symposium arrivals, the ability of an outsider drawing my life as it was on a black board. I was sitting in the back of an aisle seat left side of the room. I could have snuck out without anyone noticing but it was as if my body was magnetized to the metal folding chair. I could not budge. I wanted to know as the realist in me and at the same time wanted to escape the dreadfully brutal arrows piercing my body with every word he spoke, every chalk mark he made. In that moment all lightning bolts reverberated through me. No one else seemed effected by the recently developed revelation he was sharing. Was this possibly the overflow chamber everyone else had to go to because all the other lecture rooms were full and there was no available seating?

Still in one fever I felt myself go limb tingling numb, shocked by the wind being knocked out of me in my stationary position, as my heart sank into a desperate sadness. In that split second seemingly lasting a very long time and despite of it or perhaps because of it, my soul awakened to yet another Enlightening moment, while my mind was doing it's very best wrestling with a crumb of relief in knowing the possibility of truth.

He was a young, curly dark haired, very handsome Neurosurgeon from Boston vocalizing the newest research regarding hypothyroidism, meningioma brain tumors, the hormone estrogen and fertility. He was articulate, well spoken, and glaringly drawing my life story as if he had lived it with me, while concurrently erasing my life dreams on the chalk board. He drew the connecting dot archway from hypothyroidism, the hormone estrogen straight way to a meningioma brain tumor through to the reality of "infertility" as in never being able to carry a baby full term.

Q: Please explain the connection between hypothyroidism, meningioma brain tumors and infertility?

A: Hypothyroidism is often the result of radiation of the thyroid. The thyroid, being the thermostat of the body, controls reproduction. Low ovulation is often a symptom of hypothyroidism as is a high risk of miscarriage.

Meningiomas are sometimes a result of hypothyroidism. If the tumor is near the site of the pituitary it again adds to the difficulties of pregnancy. Meningioma patients have a higher risk of miscarriage, but the hypothyroidism is easy to treat with just a small pill taken daily that is very easy to tolerate, so, if it is detected it should be very treatable.

The tears welling up somehow simultaneously pushed down getting caught in my throat. The welling up and the pushing down were about to open the flood gates of my eyes. While I was relieved to have answers with a new burst of joyful reflection, *Now we know where to start from and where to go from here,* at the same time The Evil Twin of Joy was dashing my Spirit with the brooding judgement, *There is nowhere to go from here. You're stuck. You are that picture. No babies for you. Period. Shhhhh...* Perhaps now I had the reason. Perhaps now we had the arsenal of wisdom to move forward in our Baby Questing as we called our journey (Never did call it Infertility. That's a mind blowing, heart wrenching set-up).

Yet as if a prayer, I have never let go of the black board illustration of my life a total stranger, one who knew more than me about my life at that time, created that day in front of countless others who never knew he was painting a picture of me.

What I have learned is how much our experience still hurts sometimes. Yet each new piece of information concerning our baby quest and the loss of our dear beloved babies helps toward understanding the physical "why". It does not always calm the initial feeling of "it is my fault" nor the tears that result even though I do know better.

Many years ago during our time of Baby Making while struggling with brain tumors the medical field did not know what it knows now leading to the fact there were not as many options as there are today. Our first baby, a girl, was naturally conceived three years after my craniotomy. We were elated! Tragically our sweet infant passed this life through a miscarriage during our first trimester. We continued our quest through 2 IVF's and 3 IUI's. Our first little boy was conceived through our first IUI. We watched his heartbeat to the rhythm of our love on ultrasound. Then one day his little heart stopped beating during our first trimester. Our love ached with a desperate, tender grief.

Our second little boy was conceived during our second and last IVF. We saw him, tiny and sweet there on the screen. And then we didn't. He disappeared. He was gone. He had reabsorbed into my body during our first trimester. In those times there was breath robbing sorrow. Yet we knew during the seasons of our babies' short visits, there was a jubilation we would never have experienced had they not peeked in. We are Heaven Blessed with their presence, their love, their wisdom and joy forever and a day. Our sweet Kaily Rebecca, Joshua Gabriel and little Christopher Michael specifically choose us for a moment in time before deciding to remain in Spirit.

How did we survive all of this, brain tumors, babies, surgeries, devastating loss, together and still intact? Pure, deep, long before this lifetime abiding Soulful love and courage, lots of courage.

The following are a few well documented research papers and resources. Get yourself a cup of tea, breath in, breath out and read yourself into believing, "If this baby dream is truly mine then it is truly mine to make it come true." Do your homework physically, emotionally, mentally and spiritually. Read, read and read some more. Pray, pray and pray some more. Be present. Be clear. Find real doctors, your neurosurgeon who will tag team with your reproductive endocrinologist, both who are wise, compassionate and love making dreams come true. Then if your heart dances and your soul says "Yes," go for the teething ring!

1. *Fertility Options | American Brain Tumor Association www.abta. org › Treatment and Care Side Effects and their Management*

   "Learn about fertility options from the American Brain Tumor Association. Discover our resources on the fertility concerns and solutions after a brain tumor treatment."

2. *American Brain Tumor Association Webinar Fertility Concerns for the Brain Tumor Survivor December 11, 2013 * Dr. Lisa Kolp, OB/GYN John Hopkins University Hospital*

3. *Why do meningiomas grow during pregnancy? --ScienceDaily https://www.sciencedaily.com/ releases/2012/11/121120121813.htm* "**Meningiomas** are relatively common, usually benign (noncancerous) **tumors** that arise in the tissues lining the **brain** (meninges). They cause problems when they grow large enough to affect **brain** functions. Over the years, there have been several reports of **meningiomas** enlarging or becoming symptomatic during **pregnancy**."

4. *Fast-Growing Meningioma in a Woman Undergoing Fertility Treatments https://www.hindawi.com/journals/ crinm/2016/3287381/ by A Patterson - 2016 - Related articles Dec 7, 2016 -* "Furthermore, the patient was also taking exogenous progesterone as part of the fertility treatment as well. ... It will also expose patients to high risks of neurological deficit from both rapid tumor growth and from surgical treatment of such giant meningiomas."

FYI

American Brain Tumor Association Webinar
Fertility Concerns for the Brain Tumor Survivor
December 11, 2013
Dr. Lisa Kolp, OB/GYN John Hopkins University Hospital

Q: What about the effects of Brain MRIs
and Gamma Knife Surgery?

A: *MRIs are perfectly safe in that area although the contrast often used is not. Gamma Knife Surgery is a very high dose of radiation although focused and directed to a very specific area of the brain, the tumor itself.*

Being it is a very high dose of radiation it is a higher risk.

Little Stories — Big Memories
Marvels In Recovery Mode

Coughing Up My Lungs and Throwing Up My Toes

We had hopefully outlived the possibly of going to die although it had once again become a scary notion for us. During my hospital stay I had contracted something that was horrible and as yet undiagnosed. I was blown up like the Michelin Man to the extent of not being able to put my arms down by my side, with an outrageous rash all over my body, coughing up my lungs, throwing up my toes, both of which hurt my precious half-bald head immensely. I was very ready to blow this popsicle stand for fear of fast expiring. *I'll be damn if I'm gonna die of some kind of cooties after surviving major brain surgery,* I thought to myself. Three weeks after leaving the hospital and five docs later Mom's dermatologist looked at me entering his office doorway and asked; "Are you on Dilantin?". That would be "Yes." "Well, this is a Dilantin allergic reaction." He then took a stethoscope to my chest. "Polly, she's got double pneumonia." Off Dilantin...on to Tegretol. Drinking lots of hot lemon water, taking Bumex and being very gentle with myself.

No Knife Involved

Once able to be up and out of bed for a few minutes at a time, I was hungry to help in gratitude for my parents generous "Stay here in our home" offer. There must be something I can do. I wandered into the kitchen. My mom always created the most delightfully delectable, yummy dishes every mealtime, so often you would find her in the kitchen. I have no memory of what in particular she was sowing the seeds of that day, but it involved mushrooms. I learned a wonderful thing that day about mushrooms from my Mom. They peel! That thin skin cloaking them from what I have heard to be dirt and pig shit they grow in can be peeled away along with the dirt and pig shit. Awesome! "Honey, here, you peel the mushrooms" and she placed the plate of darkened white caps and an empty bowl in front of me at the breakfast table by the front window. I can do this. Mom kept a stealth eye on me thankful there was no knife involved. My smile beamed with the pure essence of accomplishment. I'm peeling mushrooms. Nothing to skywrite a note or slap on your back bumper like "My Child Is An Honor Student and Peels Pig Shit Off Mushrooms" but hey, this child's first job with no knife involved was peeling mushrooms just a few short weeks after major brain surgery.

What a Team

Every two hours on the dot my mom would help me up and set me out on the dining room run for health and well-being. Her dining room table easily sat thirty for a holiday feast. During our stay at my parents' home it had become my raceway. Bunny rabbit slippers shuffling through the guest bedroom, out into and through the foyer, eventually I reached the dining room where Mom was waiting. She did look rather proud of herself being part of my continuous health revival. As it should be. And so it was while Mom slipped into the adjoining kitchen where she could peek out now and then while producing one of her magnificent trays of lasagna lovingly through her Celtic heart and hands, I began my circular low speed motion around their banquet table. She alone, and along when sisters were visiting, would give a "Woo-Woo-Woo" and the cheering section wave of encouragement with each lap of achievement. The first week was an exhausting 40 minutes of touching, holding and counting 30 chairs. The next week 30 minutes and the next 20. By Christmas she was actually trusting me to plunk ice into the 30 glasses at each table setting. That's a PT walk and a balancing hold. Progress and lasagna made. What a team.

His Soulful Eyes

There is a photograph my brother Michael took Christmas Day 1989 in front of my parent's Christmas Tree that is most assuredly one of my all-time forever favorites of Kenny and me. Most people when they see it go "Ahh, that's a cute picture of the two of you." When I look at it, I see our Souls. What people don't realize looking at the image is Kenny is literally holding me up and steady. Look at our hands. I am bald on the right side of my head. Look at the slant of the bow in my hair. I am blissfully alive. Look at the Light radiating across my face. And Kenny, Kenny, is my Hero. Look in his eyes, his deeply loving compassionate Soulful eyes. I love that photo of us. Thank you, Michael, for snapping a shot of Soul.

Funny, Funny, Funny Dad

While working on that eye-hand-brain coordination thing, one of my daily single-minded practices while sitting on the floor in Dad's den, was eyeing up the placement, height and width of the room's door frame out into the foyer. I then readied myself and Peppie, Mom and Dad's little high energy Yorkie, my physical therapist assistant in tiny puppy form, for yet another run in my quest of throwing the ball through the large opening in the wall. The test: coordinating what the brain sees with what the eye's see while they hopefully communicate in collaboration with arm and hand. Peppie would then passionately retrieve the orb eagerly running it back slime-encrusted, drop it in my lap, sit high and poised, psyched for his next "Do it again" run. Picking up, handling the ball, eye-hand-brain aiming and throwing through the wide-open space was the goal to be achieved. *I can do this* was my mantra. No matter how perfectly I envisioned the connection between door frame, space, aim and trajectory, inevitably as little Peppie ran with long hair blowing on the raceway, with my prism sight, the ball continually hit instead one of Dad's honorable medical certificates lining the side of the walls with a bam and a shake. One evening as I took up my perch and readied for aim, I noticed the bare walls. "Funny, funny, funny Dad". Snug in his comfy green velvet Dad chair behind the shielding newspaper with only lap and legs exposed I hear, "Just protecting my property."

6-17-90

Dearest Dad,

More love a father could not show his child than what you have given me this past year.

You took over for me when I was frozen with fear while carrying your own fears inside. You did not rest until you knew deep within, you had found "the best in the best environment" for your baby girl. I don't think you truly rested until long after I was in your home being cared for by you.

As long as I live and eternally, I will always remember your late-night kiss goodnight and your hand, your beautiful, courageous hand on my shoulder in recovery. The Tuesday after surgery grinning that smile only you have, you held me while I cried telling me "this is normal." You really did make it all better when you told me that. Then you held onto me as I held onto you taking my longest walk to date down the G.W. hallway.

Once home, every morning, every night you came to check in on me. Sometimes while in a fog sleep, I could feel your presence before you would leave for work. I had had an especially painful, sleepless night and your peeking in always comforted and blanketed me in warmth.

The nights by the fire watching T.V. with you and Peppie are forever fond memories.

Forever I will cherish my time with you and Mom as a blessing, a unique, wonderful blessing, God gave to me. God gave to me the most wonderful, kind, generous, strong man He could create to be my father.

You may not say much, you may not show a lot of emotion, it's subtly and it's quiet that usually teaches life's finest lessons. Thank you for the many chapters of lessons you have added to my book of life.

With all my heart I thank you, I thank God, I thank Mom, for you being my Dad.

I love you so dearly, Gena - Your Brain Child
(sorry about the ticket, Pops)

Thank You Very Much

6-17-90

...rather could
...this child than
...that you have given me this
past year.
You took over for me when I
was frozen with fear while carrying
your own fears inside. You did not rest
until you knew deep within, you had found
"the best in the best environment" for your
baby girl. I don't think you truly realized
until long after I was in your home being
cared for by you. As long as I live and
eternally I will always remember; your
late night kiss goodnight and your hand,
your beautiful, courageous hand on my shoulder
in recovery - the Tuesday after surgery
grinning that smile only you have. You had
me while I cried telling me "this is
normal". you really did make it all better
when you told me that- then you held on to
me as I held onto you taking my longest
walk to date down the C.N. hallway;
Once home, every morning, every
night you came to check in on me
sometimes while in a log sleep I could
feel your presence before you could leave
for work. I had had an especially painful,
sleepless night and your teasing is always
comfort too and blanketed me in warmth.
The nights by the fires watching T.V. with

The Magical Mystery Tour of the Brain

"Hey Doc, How is it I know every word to every Beatle's song but sometimes looking right at their faces, I do not know the names of my own family members, nor do I have memory of past life changing events with Kenny, family and/or friends? No recollection at all. What part of the brain are the Beatles in?" He just laughed. "I didn't go near that part of your brain."

Pure Pleasure Indeed

Once really home, our home, rewiring the athletic brain-legs connection my daily sojourn was our quarter mile driveway from our little farmhouse to Willow Lake's gravel road. The normal three-minute walk took me 45 minutes up and after a breath break, another 45 minutes back. What I remember was the supreme joy of being able to walk enriched by the extra-ordinary particulars one misses when running the same road with purpose of just running the same road or even more so by driving to get from here to there. There were bird fellowships in song and fancy flight to be seen. Leaves and trees in landscape from the audience side of life as they danced in the breeze. Sky to adore with colors and clouds as they too moved along in their unhurried journey. As I had become a regular in their daily rounds, particular chipmunks, cats, skunks and foxes watched for me setting their time of day to this new addition in their routine. For me the freshness of air, the palatable breeze upon my face, the sights and sounds of this part of an hour and half of my day was pure pleasure indeed.

Search and Rescue

One beautiful spring day, Kenny was heading out, all geared up ready to take on the duty of lawn care. "So you are going out to..." Wait for it.... Looking for it.... *The word that means: shorten-all the same length-it will look really pretty-green-vroom-vroom-push-makes noise*...Searching the files. Found it! "You're going outside to vacuum!" "That's right, Dear. I am going outside to vacuum" he said with I'm not sure why a smirk. "Then you are going to..." This one calls for motion-brain-search communication activating the right arm into double circles, one larger than the other, round and round. "You're going to..." Looking for it... Flip the files.... Sounds like... *Make it pretty-go round and round-making circles-up against the edge-trim-straight-finish and complete*... "Cool whip! That's it! You are going outside to vacuum and cool whip!" "That's right Honey, I'm going outside to vacuum and cool whip. When I'm done I shall return from my lawn care duties of vacuuming and cool whipping." Well, I was all a smile and ever so proud of myself having accomplished a successful search and rescue wordsmith mission.

"Stop Asking or You Will Lose It"

Numbers, since my craniotomy I can do numbers. How glorious to be able to do numbers. Before brain surgery I was always afraid of numbers. It seemed I always got them wrong whether incorporating my fingers for the final count or working pencil to paper. Now suddenly I can do numbers. How very awesome to just be able to know the answer without even searching for it, no need counting digits, or getting out the eraser. The answers are just there. Now, mind you, pun intended, I am not talking about genius mathematical query. I am talking everyday numbers stuff that most take for granted but that I feared with avengeance. Now, there's the question and without a thought, seriously, without a thought, the calculation has been completed and bada-bing, here is your answer. Amazing! Wonderful! Delightful! More than just ordinary fun. How is this possible? How is this all of a sudden happening? What part of my brain is this from that may have been somehow manipulated creating this new magnificent achievement in my life? I've got to know! Looking for it...Scouring the field...Searching the files... Exploring the terrain...Analyzing it. Once that word, analyzing, came into the equation I heard strong and definitively the voice of Elizabeth, my Guardian Angel since birth, say, "Stop asking or you will lose it!" "What? Why?" "Stop asking or it will go away. You don't need to know everything." Hands up, the moment is calling for an immediate response, "You got it." Never have I again questioned this new, magical ability I have to be an ordinary math making genius person. It just is and I am totally amazed at the extra-ordinary marvel of it all.

Kenny's Six-Month Melt-Down

Windows opened with the nighttime country air of May breezing through our bedroom we were both calming our bodies down for a good night sleep. Kenny laid on his left side, eyes closed. Me nestled in supported upright by one of those pillows they call "husbands" although I'm not quite sure why being mine was right beside me. Suddenly a sound. At first, I thought it had come from outside. It was a reverberation so deep it seemed bought up from middle earth. Again, the shatter in silence. Quickly I realized it was a sigh, a giant exhale emitting from Kenny. The titan out breath was followed by heartbreaking sobs. He turned over onto his back placing himself in a better position for his body to let go. "Kenny, Honey, what's wrong?" He could barely catch his breath. Allowing the moment for him to do so he answered, "I think I'm just beginning to realize what I've been through with you in the last six months." Finally, finally, his turn to let go and give himself the space to crumble. His left arm over my body, his right arm hugging my back, he lay his head in my lap and wept. All I could do is stroke his hair and quietly thank him for all he had been while navigating through the strange terrain of brain surgery with his Beloved. Finally exhausted and softly falling asleep from his well-deserved six month melt down, he whispered, "Brain surgery has stolen our innocence." I held my breath as my eyes focused into the realm of a different kind of understanding, complete love and devotion from his point of view.

My right hand cradling his head, my left laying upon his back, it must have been an hour or so before his body freed itself from the tension of release resuming its natural rhythmic flow of breath. Finally rest, real baby like rest. My body and mind sighed a silent weeping. "Good night my Sweet Prince. Please accept my apology. I love you."

Chapter Four

Again With The Brain Tumor
This Side of Life

Seventeen Years Later
I Can't, I Just Can't

"Katherine, I can't! I just can't! I can't take him back there again!" Clearly, I should have pulled over as I was weeping so intensely, I could hardly see through the windshield of my own eyes none the less the actual windshield of my Toyota, but I was in a flaming flurry to get out. Get out of DC, get out of the crowd of drivers on New York Avenue as it felt like they were crushing me, get out of this I can't believe this is happening again nightmare, get out of me, my head. Get out, just get out! This time I was not only scared, I was confused and angry. I had not been angry last time, not even a little bit. So this was painful in and of itself as I rarely do anger. It's too, well, angry a feeling for me to deal with. I'd rather bypass it and go to the real feeling behind it and that is usually hurt, but how do you get to being hurt about having a brain tumor... again. Who or what hurt you? It wasn't like I was angry at God. It wasn't God who hurt me. That just seems stupid to me. So, was I angry at the tumor? I don't want to be angry at the tumor! It's inside me! I don't want to be angry at something inside me! That seems rather counter productive. Yet the anger was real. And I just knew, I couldn't take Kenny back there again, back into the brain tumor reality. I just can't!

Two of my check points on how my brain is doing were outside their lines of my normalcy. Finding words and doing numbers had become challenging again and headaches were becoming too frequent for comfort. I knew my blessed brain was not oaky.

Usually I schedule my MRI's and Dr. Kobrine visits on a sentimental memory day. I know, goofy. What's sentimental about an MRI or a visit to your neurosurgeon? Life, life is sentimental about an MRI and daily blessings are attributed at least in part to my neurosurgeon. Had I not had the first MRI and met Dr. Arthur Kobrine when I did in the history of my life, I would not be here now. They are magic, marvelous and awesomely wonderful in the good that they do. So, to relieve the scary, anxious part of not so happy possibilities connected with them, I honor their goodness in my calendar of Celebratory Days. October 19 was my very first MRI ever, November 7 was the day we met Dr. Kobrine and my Brain Buddy Beamer, November 16 was my craniotomy and new life begins, November 22 was the day I left the hospital alive in recovery, December 7 was my first Post-Op visit.

This wasn't any of those days. In fact, it wasn't even day. It was a winter early dark evening about 7:00 pm. I had purposefully scheduled this MRI without Kenny being present. I knew something was in there or at least I thought I knew. They, Anne Arundel Medical Hospital Center powers that be, had redesigned the Imaging Department. It was no longer the outside trailer connected by the interim little comfort cubby welcome center. The new space was cold, white-gray, bleak with the usual institutional chairs lined up against the wall awkwardly placed across from the curtained changing booths. Sitting on the very edge of the chair in what seemed to be limbo land, as it wasn't the reception area nor was it in site of the MRI capsule room, waiting for what I hoped to be just a normal scan, 'Everything looks great, Regina' was contrary to what I intuitively knew. *Oh, good, here comes Vickki.*

My very special Vickki MRI Tech all these years, seventeen years to be exact. She'll tell me the good news and all will be well again. It was just all in my head, as they say. Instead she handed me the films, eyes to the floor. Her gentle, loving voice still echoed hours later; "Go see Kobrine as soon as you can." She turned and left walking heavy, head down. She never met my eyes. Oh, My God! Vickki didn't even look in my eyes. No hug as we parted. I was frozen watching her leave me. Gone from sight, my exhale spoke my truth, *I knew it. Something is wrong.*

I had the films up on the light table before Doc Arthur entered the room. He entered in silence. Not meaning too but as the door opened his eyes caught sight of the images on the wall straight across from him. I think that's when the silence versus hello hug caught him. "What the hell? Why is that there?" He came close enough to the viewing as if to confront it face to face. "It's not the same tumor but it is another tumor. I don't get it. Why would that happen all these years later? I don't get it." "You don't get it? You don't know why? It's in my head and I don't get it."

"Okay, this time I want you to go see Dr. Ladislau Steiner in Charlottesville. We'll do Gamma- Knife." *Ah, that's comforting. A sentence regarding my head with the word knife in it. I feel better already.* "Why him? Why Gamma Knife, whatever that is? Why not you? I want you." "Dr. Ladislau Steiner is one of the inventors of Gamma Knife and he is right here in Charlottesville, Virginia." That is about the last I heard in this conversation. What I had heard was, 1. I had another brain tumor, 2. I needed surgery, 3. Dr. Kobrine wasn't going to do it, 4. I had to go away to have it done, 5. Knife was in the same sentence, 6. Blah, Blah, Blah, Blah, 7. I had another brain tumor, 8. I needed surgery, 9. Dr. Kobrine wasn't going to do it, 10. I had to go away, 11. Knife, Brain, Gamma, 12. *I can't, I just can't tell Kenny...*Wow! When had I slipped from hearing outside myself to the circle of words being created inside my head?

Now, in the car and driving. Driving home? Driving where? Where do I go to be safe with this news about me and what I needed to do or at least decide what I am going to do? I can't go home. Kenny's there. I can't take him back there again. Who can I trust right here, right now, to talk to that won't tell a soul, who won't tell Kenny? Katherine! My little, tiny toy person, Reiki Master-Teacher, Soul Sister, Katherine. I can trust Katherine. Oh, good, whip her with the news, depend heavy on her for keeping the secret from my Beloved who happens to be her friend as well. That's not fair yet I found myself dialing her number on my cell phone. "KJ, do you have a minute?"

Our conversation was long and very weepy on my end of the phone. Katherine stood strong and soft in her voice, never wavering, her usual mastership. "I hear what you are saying, Regina. I will keep your secret, but I really think you need to tell Kenny. He is strong. Yes, I will most assuredly go with you, but I really think you need to reconsider telling Kenny. He would want to know." "Katherine, I can't. I just can't. I can't take him back there again. He went through it last time and it's just too much to ask. It's not fair to him. He didn't ask for this!" "Neither did you, Regina."

Cindy Kobrine, Dr. Kobrine's wife and Office Manager, called with preferred dates for my consult appointment and day of Radio-Surgery. *Radio-Surgery? That's a weird word. Was I going to be able to tune in, change channels and hear my inner thoughts out loud for the rest of my life after this procedure?* The tuning in and changing channels was a welcome thought but the out loud was a bit unnerving. *Was everybody else going to be able to tune in, change channels and hear me walking down the road or in the aisles of the supermarket? How does this Radio-Surgery work?* I started doing my internet homework and my novice sheet of unlimited questions began. Still, I did not say a thing to Kenny. I just could not imagine sharing this news and taking him down this road again. In 1989 first time ever having to face the world of brain tumor, surgery, recovery and all it entailed, he not once left my side. I had heard me say more than once, "I don't know which would be worse, to be the person with the brain tumor or to be the person who loved the person with the brain tumor." I watched and at times felt what he went through as good as he was at allowing it all to pass through him nearly un-effected. Continually like a broken record I heard myself repeat, *I just cannot take him back there again. It's not fair.* So, I was planning a secret, 'Just us Girls, Honey', brain surgery trip to Charlottesville, Virginia with Katherine all the while knowing how crazy that all sounds. I had not a clue what this all would entail. What my head would look like and how I would explain it if it were crazy wild head shave cut. What was recovery going to be? How long would we be gone? Could I really pull this off without Kenny being involved? Could I really go do this and then just come home never in all our life say a thing about it and he would never, ever know? That's just crazy with a near demented twist in my way of doing us. We tell each other everything always.

Weeks went by without my saying anything. Katherine continued to keep my secret with her in breath all the while gently swaying me to share the news with Kenny with her out breath. "I will still go with you. It can still be just me and you, Regina, and I encourage you to tell Kenny. He would want to know."

Finally, I caved. I wasn't doing this keeping something from Kenny so very well as it had never been done before. He "already knew something was up and was just waiting for me to be ready to share it".

Of all days to surrender, it was New Year's Day 2007. "Kenny, Honey, I have something to tell you. Something I don't want to tell you ...I have another...And it's called Gamma Knife...And Katherine is going with me so you don't even have to go...So, it's all arranged... And we're going to go...And " And the "And's" stopped as Kenny put his finger up against my lips while drawing my body in close for one of his mighty man hugs wrapped in adoring devotion and affectionate compassion. The hug where one of his hands is caressing the back of my heart as if our bodies have melded into one and the other cradling the back of my skull like a baby's butt, giving me no reasonable doubt I am safe and protected in comfort, love and joy. I could feel his heart beating against the outward body of my chest entering into my bodies heart cavity as his words whispered through every cell of my being, "Katherine can go with us if she wants to." My body submitted through total collapse to our need never to keep a truth from each other as it would lead to lying for the rest of our life.

The rest of the day was often clothed in silence. While I spent most of the day nestled in the corner of our sofa sitting crossed legged weeping from time to time cuddling Asti, our tiny Soul Puppy Yorkie, Kenny catered to my needs radiating strength, wonder and "Katherine can go with us if she wants to." I couldn't help but think, *Happy New Year, Babe, and guess what, I've got another brain tumor.* Yet I felt stronger now and ready for the journey to come. We're gonna do this and it will be done from a place of higher knowing having been through it once already. We will prepare our healthy bodies, calm emotions, peaceful minds and glorious spirits believing all will be well because it will. "Katherine, I told Kenny."

Gamma Wizard

The very moment we entered The University of Virginia Hospital Medical Center in Charlottesville, Virginia we could tell it was different from the traditional hospital med hub. There was a brilliance about it that could be seen and felt. There was a spaciousness that exuded comfort and peace. The customary hospital white was a different white than the predictable. This white was radiating a Light of healing. I'm not quite sure how they did that from the simplicity of paint on the walls and shiny under footings. And "it" was clear, the atmosphere, the aura, the air, was clear of the usual thick goopiness of attached illness. Everywhere was clean beyond the sweeping and mopping of floors. It was an invitation to one's own healing.

The nice lady behind the reception desk shared a tenderness from her heart just in how she answered the question I'm sure she hears over and over during her day, "How do we get to...". Our how do we get to, was the Brain Tumor Lars Leksell Gamma Knife Radio-Surgery Center. *No, not Ginsu, Gamma,* I heard my silly voice say inside my head. It all seemed very silly in a way. Leaving home, leaving our puppy Asti with a friend, traveling miles and hours down the road, walking into a place unknown to our comfort zone, asking about a Gamma Knife Department as if asking how to get to the Home Decor Department of an anchor store in the Mall.

Following her direction, we walked down the bright hallway. A foyer with plants and large windows allowing one to see there is a world, a beautiful world, outside a hospital confinement. This entranceway led to a tunneling corridor which led to a staircase with only one direction, down. The white walls were now gray. As in matter? Did they do that on purpose? Were they truly that conscious? Everything seemed done with an intentional awareness here. I'm not sure how many turns it took but it literally spiraled seemingly for quite a distance and with every new leading coil the staircase itself narrowed. At the bottom stood a large double door. I remember turning to Ken remarking,

"I believe we have hit Middle Earth." Later in our brief journey the metaphor of Middle Earth and the procedure known as Gamma Knife took on a completeness in its understanding. It was all so perfect.

Entering through the doors was like walking onto the set of a sci-fi movie. Everything was very white, compartmentalized, glassed in, and sterile yet in a welcoming way. I'm not sure how they pulled that one off, but they did and they did it well. There were libraries of this and that. Books, big reels of film, MRI files, all behind big glass walls. There were people here and there in white lab coats, looking ever so scientific. We met the receptionist, Mary Burton, who I later deemed "His Number One." She was genuinely pleasant as she explained the paperwork to be filled out including Advance Directives and Power of Attorney.

As we had been instructed, we knew these documents were necessary to bring along with current MRI's, driver's license and insurance card. We had done our research both outward and inward before making the affirming decisions. Questions and answers that aren't as fun as what's for dinner tonight but once complete getting past the who's who to take over if Kenny is not "at one's disposal", there is a comfort and peace about having it all in place. I think it has to do with the release of burden. In so doing, one takes on the responsibility that most of the time befalls loved ones because said document is not in place. Once complete all anyone has to do is follow your guide. There is a joy in releasing others from this burden and a confidence in oneself for making the decisions about their own life such as it is in the moment.

With registration forms complete and after a few minutes of Number One checking over the facts, we were told how to navigate into Dr. Ladislau Steiner's office just through the door. One step in and I knew I was in love. There were piles, piles everywhere. On his desk, on bookshelves, on the floor and on nearly every "flat space", as Kenny calls them, that I bet under it all was possibly a six-foot table. Piles just like my office except his piles were bigger, taller, towering and somehow exuded a magnificence of other wisdom. I've heard it said piles in an office are a sign of genius. In my case, a sign of an overwhelmed, loving the work, Healing Center Director. In this exhibition, just like in my office, I/he knew where everything, every piece of paper, every article, every needed document was placed into what pile soon, one day, to be filed properly. Looking about, just like in my office, there were angel statues and paintings on this shelf and in that corner. "Kenny, I love him already." We sat briefly waiting in the two out of three chairs minus a pile.

He walked in unannounced, no fanfare. Dr. Ladislau Steiner, MD, Ph.D., Professor of Neurosurgery and Radiology, Director of Lars Leksell Center for Gamma Surgery, University of Virginia Health System, Department of Neurosurgery. He introduced himself and took our hands in a kind way before moving to his seat behind his desk. Already two things most docs don't do. They usually forget to introduce themselves as if somehow you should automatically know who they are, maybe by the way they carry themselves or some paper they wrote for a medical journal you should have read and would have seen their affixed photo. Secondly, he took our hands inviting us to touch his. His hands which would soon be working magic regarding my head and the visitor within. "So, what questions do you have for me today?" he asked in a most intriguing accent. He was from Transylvania. *Really? Seriously? The real Transylvania, as in Frankenstein. Steiner... Frankenstein- ner? Could this get any more surreal? Okay, back to this reality, Regina...* He answered every one of my questions and believe me there were a boatload. Then he added, "Here is what else you need to know." He went to one of his piles extracting a big book with articles and photos of what Gamma Knife was about, and why it would be performed, why it makes sense in my case. He passionately proceeded to another pile in another area of his office pulling out the papers and articles of how it would be performed. He was showing us his research as one of the inventors, along with Lars Leksell, of Gamma Knife Surgery, sometimes referred to as Stereotactic Radio-Surgery, although I am not quite sure why being there are no speakers, transmitters or boom boxes involved.

Did I mention he was 87 years of earth age and that he was small in his physical body and reminded me of my Dad who was also small in stature, big in doctor? Did I mention he was totally engaging in his demeanor, his ability to listen, really listen to our concerns, his passion of surgical artistry and that he loved Pollard the painter and dearly missed his wife, Melita, his life partner in heart and soul as well as professionally, Dr. Melita Steiner, who had just passed over only months earlier?

We spent a good hour and a half with him never once feeling like, he might be feeling, "It's time for you to go now." Actually, it was he who finally asked, "Any more questions? If you do just call here this afternoon, otherwise take the rest of the day off and I will see you two here bright and early tomorrow morning." He had shared every detail of the procedure with us in a language for our understanding. There would be a multitude of people in the room, including his surgical assistant and I would have my very own full-time personal nurse with me throughout the procedure giving full attention to my wakeful needs the entire time. He left the room only when he felt we were comfortable with the transaction of all questions answered, fears calmed, and as far as we could take it, spirits ready for tomorrow's procedure. Spirits ready... Somehow it was obvious to us both that we truly were in a different world having stepped through that double door. There was more happening here than meets the human eye. There were other worlds in play here both Devic and Extraterrestrial. As we left through the way we came, passing by the desk of Mary, Number One, I turned to her exclaiming, "He's a wizard!" Number One smiled a smile of inner knowing, "Why yes he is."

Kenny and I went off to explore James Madison's home place as if we were on vacation and this was part of the itinerary before heading back to our dear friend's home in Richmond where we were staying the night. There truly is something about Charlottesville, Virginia that is other worldly. It is beautiful in its small town-ness and its majestic nature and there is definitely something other worldly about it.

The next morning the alarm woke us to the day by 4:00 am. No drink, no breakfast, instead big hugs and loving kisses from our soul friends, Ken and Renee'. We were off traveling in the early morning pre-dawn dark from Richmond to Charlottesville. I couldn't help but think of our puppy Asti, who was staying with our friends, Joe and Carol, back on the Eastern Shore of Maryland. I had never left him more than a few hours at a time before. I wondered had he slept well overnight without being in our arms? Was he eating, playing, napping okay? Was he comfortable physically, emotionally, mentally and in his little giant spirit? Did he know we would be home soon?

I had readied for this day for months as if training for an athletic event on every level of being I was aware of. I wanted to do this well to be well. Shivani, a dear friend, and my Ayurvedic Physician, had been one of my guides through my preparedness. She coached me and my body in alignment with my intentions. I ate kitchari and only kitchari for weeks three times a day. She gave me hot stone massages. Of course, my meditation practice was highlighted with the visualizations of a positive outcome. Prayer was high on my list of communication. I did my homework. I was ready.

As we arrived in the stillness of dark there seemed a ring of Radiance arched over the campus of the Virginia Hospital Medical Center. Our steps became part of the encircling of the staircase, the mystical entranceway spiraling down into Gamma Knife middle earth. Once through the double doors there was light. A bright yet comforting light. We were shown a curtained stall for our pre-procedure pause. I gowned. Kenny bound by my side. Sitting on the gurney I felt a calmness surely different than other times in similar pre-op situations. We were periodically checked in on and vitals taken prior to my being slipped into a wheelchair launched for the qualifying ride toward the inner sanctum. I was remembering the phone calls to Beamer, my Brain Buddy Bookend, during her Gamma Knife procedure when she was here years earlier. She was alone, frightened and in pain on oh, so many levels. I had volunteered to go with her, but she refused saying,

"It's no big deal. I'll be home that night." That was her experience and this was mine. I was well prepared and again my Beloved was by my side making all the difference in the world, my world.

Kenny could be in the OR with me most of the time except when the Halo was being placed upon my head (Halo sounds so much better than frame) and during the actual time of Gamma Radiation being projected toward the tumors. As our hands slipped from their embrace I was wheeled further into the unknown. There seemed to be quite a few people present for the occasion. I was told later for the next six hours there were twenty-two attendants in all. I do remember faces. They were kind and bright and gentle faces. Each person was considerate in their interaction and communication with me. "I am Greg Patterson. I will be your nurse today. "*Oh My! Nurse Eye-Candy,* I smiled quietly to myself. Tall, at least from where I was sitting, build like a chiseled DaVinci statue as he stood arms folded in a manner to bulge his biceps, legs planted grounding the earth, bald in a gentle kinda way and shiny, Spirit shiny. "Okay" is all I could think to say. My Spirit was still and calm, listening and responding to their instructions. I was just to sit there while being given a short duration of twilight anesthesia only enough to place the Halo. I would wake with it attached to my head. *Okay, kinda weird.* I'm clueless and having to completely in total faith surrender to the experience. Next thing I know I started to feel that old familiar, 'I'm going out' feeling. The one Dr. Steiner the day before called "my aura". Urgently I called Greg over, "Greg, I need an ammonia tab and I need it right now because I'm leaving. I'm leaving right now!" Greg stood firm with a gentle command in his voice, "An ammonia tab. Now. She needs it right now. She's leaving." Only seconds passed through time, yet I knew it was too late. I looked up at him, "I'm leaving, I'm gone...I..." and gone I was as I continued to hear those about me. "She's gone. Her heart has stopped."

I could somewhat feel my body but more like it was an attachment than its physicality. Suddenly his familiar and totally unique accent was heard toward the left of what was me in body and below the me I am above. "Get it on her. Get the Halo on her. She will self-resolve." There was such a calm confidence about his being present as if he knew something no one else did. I am not sure how long this episode was, but they listened, and I heard, and I was back in body with my beating heart. I woke framed. My first thought was, *"So, this is what it is like to be a wrought iron fence looking out into the world." What went wrong, if that is even the correct word or thought? I was so prepared, so ready.* "How are you feeling? You are back." His smiling face gleamed on the other side of the barricade. I don't think I answered out loud.

"You're alright. Not to worry. Kenny can come in soon." He patted my shoulder. I saw Nurse Eye-Candy standing behind and towering over him as if he were his protecting Genie, arms folded bulging those biceps. Breathe, just breathe.

News flash, I can't move. I've got a wrought iron stockade on my head and it's kinda heavy, but I could feel Kenny's presence on the right side of me and now I feel his hand in mine. For six hours, lots of folks were very busy all around me. They were calculating this and calculating that. From time to time adjusting my head ever so slightly this way and that. I could hear his Transylvania voice quietly giving commands and folks moved in unison to his request as if everyone knew their place in time and space for such an occasion. There was nothing robotic about it. It was a symphony, a dance, an artistry in motion and I was the main benefactor in place watching through a very stiff veil. At one point I remember saying to Greg, "I need my Sacred Mountain. Kenny has the oil with him. May I please just smell it?" Without a word he disappeared as if vanishing in thin air. Not surprising. Then reappearing again in front of me and my frame, it really was a frame at that point although I was hopeful my own personal Halo was shining. He then did something I would never have thought to do. Greg doused a cotton swab with the YLO Sacred Mountain, forever my surgical and Ministerial favorite, and taped it to the frame bar below my nose. Inhaling I was centering again. "Wow! What's that?", several room participants asked. "It's an oil called Sacred

Mountain. It's helping to center her." "And us", I heard one man say off to the left of my barrier vision. *Wow! They and this place truly are other worldly.* Not once did I hear, "Holy Crap! What's that? It's not alcohol. Get rid of it. Get it out of here. Now. Stat." And they all went back to their prospective duties inhaling and enjoying the moment from yet another higher perspective if at all possible, from where they already were.

"Greg, do you remember Beamer?" Beamer was the name I had given my dear Brain Buddy Bookend as she was a beam of Light. We were each other's Brain Bookend in accord to where our tumors resided, mine, right temporal lobe, hers left frontal. We figured if we put our brain's together, we would have all the wisdom in existence and could solve the world's problem's bringing peace unto the nations. My Beamer died too early for our adventure to come to fruition. In this moment I spoke her given name, Patricia Beamer O'Sullivan, for familiarity purposes. "I do. She was a Light." "She and I were on the phone during her Gamma Knife. She was up and walking about. Is that normal? Do most people do that?" "Yes, that is the norm." "Why can't I do that? I know I can't but why?" "Regina, you are not most people, you are not the norm."

Kenny was with me a lot that day in the same room right beside me. Only when the Gamma, Cobalt Radiation Rays, four hundred forty-four, as I was told, two tumors, double shot, were coming through directed pointedly at the tumors was there no one in the room. I remember the exodus from time to time once all the computations were complete, my head angled, all set and at Dr. Steiner's command there was a hushed whooshing sound as all left. "Hello, anybody here?" I would hear his voice over the intercom, "We're all here, Regina".

At one point during the hush of readiness, as each white coat participant did what they were there to do in their part of the plan, I glanced over at Greg to my right through my partition railing. I raised my right hand ever so slightly, seeing it as if it were a separate entity on the other side of my enclosure similar to an animation. Waving my seemingly automated cupped fingers I motioned a gentle summons, "Come." Greg was now close enough for my intentional whisper, "You do know you are from the Devic Kingdom, don't you?", I asked somehow knowing he would completely understand the question without weird connotation. "No, I'm not. I'm Jinn." He then pulled himself into the background towering overall, his eyes alert to every energetic wave, arms folded, biceps bulging, holding sacred space, owning time, seemingly eclipsing over us all. My eyes, my brain, my spirit simultaneously was illuminated with an inner connection between our souls. *Oh My God! He totally gets it! He really is. This place truly is other worldly and everyone here knows it! I am, my Life Force, is totally and completely safe in their care. I truly do have a Genie in physical form of a nurse caring for me.*

Six hours later, all the glitter of Cobalt Blue gathered in my head, all the good of God's work done, the miracle of Gamma Knife was complete by my very own Gamma Wizard of its Co-Creation. Still everyone seemed to have the same exhilarating energy they came in with nearly half a day's time earlier. Their faces beamed a brightness and their spirit's exuded loving care. Time for Regina to be returned to her physical form minus the wrought iron fencing. The Halo was to be released.

Why are we getting out the Craftsman tool from Sears electric screwdriver? *Okay, that was a weird sensation on the back of my head. Ah, screws...there really are screws in my head keeping this thing on. Bride of Franken...Ouch!* I can still hear the sound of in-out-in-out-forward-reverse-forward-reverse and feel the slight sensation accompanying the pull and tug. "Doctor, this one is stuck." *I have a screw stuck in my head?* Sure enough, there was a screw stuck and tangled in my hair left forehead. At that point Dr. Ladislau Steiner could have left the room as most doctors would have at the end of a surgical procedure expecting their cronies to finish picking up the pieces. Instead standing by my left side close enough to touch my arm he motioned instructions to his assistants as I could partially view them from where I sat still affixed in frame while other's behind held up the other side. As the gardeners of my care continued their endeavor toward my freedom of scaffolding, Dr. Steiner worked his magic in compassion.

"You are Italian. You must love wine." Left turn as my mind went elsewhere from where it was. "No, you don't want to see me on that. I'm a cheap date." "Well, I have a bottle of wine in my office for a special occasion and now I know why I have been saving it. I'm going to go get it and put it in your IV and we will just see what happens." My heart felt an opening of joy as I realized what he was doing. He was just like my Dad. He could have left the OR. His purposeful work was done. He could have said, "You take care of it. My work here is done." Instead there he stood by my side, his hand on my shoulder, doing his very best to distract me from the pain involved of having a screw stuck in my head. His compassionate love overflowed the universe in that moment. He truly loved his patients. His life work truly was his dharma and if you were going to be in his presence you were to become a part of it without fail. He was a God inspired Wizard. Ahhh, the weight of the helmet lifted, pain released, I only remember a smile forming across my face and all of those beaming back at me who were now clapping at days end honoring the completion of our heroic challenge, the fight for my brain's healing. "I will still have that bottle of wine in my office waiting special for you."

Usually at this time there is a recovery period and folks are released to go home. Because "Regina, you are not the norm" occurred earlier that day, I was instead admitted into the hospital for overnight observation and neurological evaluation the following day. Before heading to the elevator there was the fitting of a heart monitor Dr. Steiner insisted upon. I laid upon the gurney while two attendees, who were among the OR entourage, did their very best to fit a working heart monitor upon me. I considered myself a post procedure lucky girl as one was most definitely Mr. Easy On The Eyes while the other was a young light loving heart, a tailored, well-mannered James Dean type in a white coat with a smile to melt by. Meanwhile the two of them were becoming quite perplexed as each heart monitor, three in all, they connected would stop it's work once it was laid upon me. "It was just working", my very own personal James Dean would say confused. "Test it over on the counter. It really was just working." It's true. It worked its heart monitor magic plugged in over on the counter. "Okay, let's try this one", Easy Eyes suggested. It, too, worked just fine on the countertop but once attached to me, nada. "I don't get it. It's working over there but not over here. There's another one in the room next door. I know it's working just fine. I just used it. How 'bout go get that one and we'll use it" a bewildered JD suggested.

Should I tell these boys, it's not the monitor, it's me? It's me and electrical things. "Um, guys, it's not the monitors. It's me." "I knew it" declared Doc JD, as if in on a kindred secret. "I knew it was you. When you were wheeled into the OR, I saw the Light surrounding you. I have never seen such a huge surrounding Light as the One you carry with you." Baby Blue Eyes just smiled as if his heart were going to break out laughing.

"Meanwhile, after what happened earlier today, we've got to get a heart monitor on you to transport you up to your room." Both gentlemen looked about them, looked back at me, and each other coming to simultaneous smirks upon their faces. "Okay, we could be here a very long time trying monitor after monitor and it's still not going to get you upstairs on a working one. Here's the deal" Mr. Easy Eyes turned Sneaky Pete said under his breath. "I'm going to lay this one on your chest as if it is operating properly, you are not going to leave us and we'll make it look like all is well as we transport you up to your room getting you settled upstairs. Okay?" "Works for me." I whispered with a grin. "Okay, here we go." The three of us traveled the halls and elevator with our allied secret inner smile of wisdom keeping our three-way trade coded confidentiality unknown to the rest of the world. Once in the room and my body transferred to the bed, my bodyguard boys both gave a sigh of "we made it" relief.

Kenny was already in the room waiting. He seemed a little concerned about the time it took us to get there maybe thinking something went awry. His wrinkled brow gave way to happy eyes once I rolled into the room. My memory of the night is foggy except for moments of slight uncomfortable wakefulness and facial views of Kenny and my brother Michael. My brother Michael, another family nurse, lived somewhat close by in Virginia and made the trek down to check in on me, us. Finding me admitted knowing I was lying in a single not double Hyatt bed he did his best to find a comfortable apparatus to pull into the same room for Ken's rest beside me. A sweet gesture of kindness and then he was gone.

Early the next morning the door opened and in walked tiny giant Dr. Steiner with his ever-present Genie Greg standing in guard behind him. My personal Jinn Nurse's face was stern, but his eyes told the story of a gentle heart. "How are you feeling today?" Dr. Steiner inquired. "I am sending you for testing today..." he went on. "I know you know best, but shouldn't we give my brain a bit of a rest being it was jumbled about quite a bit yesterday. Having been through a lot, it may not show it's best today." "That is the time to test it."

The Neurologist, Dr. Mark Quigg, MD, was such a Neuro Geek. I swear he is the person of honor the world of characters based Where's Waldo after. Upon our first meeting he was all black or white, no in-between, no other possibilities but what showed on the graph. Yet that day after my EEG, speaking with him regarding the difference on my graphed activity between a seizure and a gifted vision he was brave to say, "I don't know anything about that." I could only respond with, "I love you." He is honest, forthright and daring enough to study other than what his profession dictates. Over the next two years he, Kenny and I delighted one another with outside the box possibilities of other realities that just may not be normally accounted for on medical testing charted graphs.

Each person who touched our lives during those days at the University of Virginia Medical Hospital Center in Charlottesville, Virginia was unique in their abilities, kind in their interactions, compassionate beyond the usual white coat education. I am convinced on some level each had to submit their Spiritual Journey Resume along with the usual employment paperwork upon entry for consideration of service to humanity.

Still we are in awe to have been with Dr. Ladislau Steiner, the magnificent, compassionate Wizard who Co-Created the invention of Gamma Knife RadioSurgery, a non-invasive brain procedure. Being in his presence was a Blessing from The Hierarchy we carry with us daily. Still to this day, we are affixed in life to my personal Genie Greg, our friend connected in heart and soul.

To all others that day, while I do not remember all their names, I do have a very clear memory of their faces and the Light shining through their eyes. A great gratitude is felt for Dr. Arthur Kobrine who sent us to another worldly place for Heavenly work to be done for the survival of my brain, body and soul intact. The possible outcome of Gamma Knife Surgery as Dr. Steiner shared with us was: 1. To dissolve the tumors all together, 2. To arrest their growth, 3. To shrink the tumors and/or, 4. There would be no change at all.

Door Number 3: The meningioma tumors within my brain shrunk slightly over the first four years after Gamma Knife RadioSurgery. Now and still to this day they are behind Door Number Two, in sleeping mode. Shhhhhhhh....

Chapter Five

Just A Thought — In a Moment
June 8, 2007
Just A Thought — All Day Everyday Miracles
July 20, 2007
Just A Thought — Lessons To Be Learned
November 9, 2007

Articles from the Record Observer

Written by Rev. Regina Maria Cross

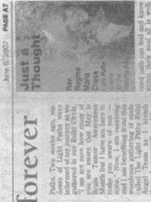

Just a Thought

Rev. Regina Maria Cross

Record Observer

COMMUNITY

In a moment, a life is changed forever

In a moment, a life is changed forever

From the Record Observer, Page A7
June 8, 2007

In one moment, life is what we assume as normal, and within a flash, all of life is different, colliding with words from what sounds like a foreign language — yet are all too familiar within your vocabulary. "Looking at your most recent MRI, there is evidence that you have another brain tumor." "What did you say?"

In a flash, shock hits along with all the experience of the past. "What did you say?" I asked, knowing that symptoms had slowly, discretely appeared that even I thought perhaps it's my thyroid in testing. I don't even remember if I asked the question aloud of my longtime companion neurosurgeon Dr. Kobrine, or whether my whole being, physical, emotional, mental and spiritual disappeared into a cocoon of sheltered safety.

Oct. 19, 1989, all of life became frighteningly surreal when I first heard the statement uttered by a very excited, lacking in communications skills, doctor. "You have a brain tumor!" In a moment, life as we knew it was changed forever. A brain tumor did not figure into our year number eight of marriage, our loving pet companions, the deep longing for children, for the country house soon to be serenely surrounded by the white picket fence. The words "brain tumor" never came up in conversation.

Since that all too authentic day, through a craniotomy on Nov. 16, 1989, followed by years of subtle recovery I have sometimes felt as a stranger navigating through a strange land, sometimes full of wonder, other times totally uncoordinated. Yet having survived given less than a 20 percent chance of making it off the table, I questioned my existence having heard, felt and saw those in the hospital rooms next to me having a near full chance of recovery die.

I marvel at peripheral vision, which most people don't even think about, as it is just a part of their sight, but I hold up my hands to the sides of my head and I can see my fingers wiggle. Being able to "do numbers" when anything to do with numbers prior to diagnosis put fear in my heart yet four years later feeling as a wizard might feel, being able to remember more than one number at a time when making a phone call or working the books, eventually coming to the intuitively understood studies of Numerology. Then there is getting the fork in my mouth as aimed versus another pick to the forehead, that's big if for no other reason but social etiquette.

After seven years having what I term an "alternative thought," a process of being able to think another way, of doing something versus all is lost if not done the one way, the other way I can think it. And reading, the absolute miraculous ability of knowing what the word is, the meaning and comprehending all of them together in a sentence. (Now I write a monthly column for my town paper! Wow!).

All this daily leads to a place of walking in One's bliss and joy. A place of choosing wisely all that surrounds you in respect to the miracle being alive in life is.

Now, almost two decades later, not only do I know what I know from all these years of experience, always including the spiritual aspect of my life's journey, which is everything of it, but what about what I don't know of the upcoming procedure I will be giving myself over to later in June. How do I do this with what I know this time and what I don't?

For months since this diagnosis, I have been silent keeping the news to myself slowing sharing only when I felt comfortable, taking yet another step forward off Shocks Avenue.

Yet what am I waiting for? Who says enlightenment means never asking for help for yourself? I thought I had healed that '50s Roman Catholic, Italian female upbringing!

Within Light Paths we have co-created The Reiki Angel Team comprised of well-trained, practiced and highly intuitive student/practitioners of Traditional Reiki Natural Healing.

Weekly, one or two of us are with a dear one undergoing their time of diagnosed living invited upon their journey contracted between themselves and God (don't misunderstand me…I do not believe God gives us illness, allows it Yes, gives it No…it's called free-will).

I started thinking about what we had created, what we were doing and questioning any teaching strategy as Spiritual Director at Light Paths. Two weeks ago, students of Light Paths were informed of my journey as we gathered in our Reiki Circle. "I am not sure how many of you are aware that May is Brain Tumor Awareness Month, but I am here to make you aware of one – mine." Now, I am receiving, and I am benefiting from this wondrous gathering of souls called The Light Paths Reiki Angel Team as I breathe through preparation for a less invasive tumor treatment called Stereotactic Radiosurgery, particularly Gamma Knife (do we have to use the word knife? How 'bout Gamma Jamma, or Gamma Yeah, it just sounds lighter, happier, more conducive to healing.)

In the beginning, shock, fear and chaos pounce. Breathe, just breathe, God gave us life's breath, prana, not to stop it before our time but to breathe through the challenges we create asking for assistance from those souls incarnate at the same time, on the same planet with the same beating heart of Universal Love, the Divine Spark Within, so that in those moments of frail humanness even those on their enlightened path can feel and know within their soul all is well, even when life appears to suck.

In some moments of living, life is forever changed and the many moments that follow each of us has a choice to continue them in fear or to ask for the very reasons we are here, love and healing. God gave us each other for this very purpose and for this realization I am grateful.

For me It's Just A thought that gives me courage.

All day, every day miracles

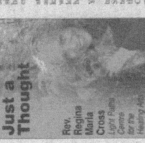

Just a Thought

Rev.
Regina
Maria
Cross

*Light Faith
Centre
for the
Healing Arts*

"Uh. Oh. Quick I need an operating table! I'm going, quick, I'm leaving"

"She's back. You got a little excitement into our day. Your heart stopped."

"Ken, during the Halo MRI we found a second brain tumor."

As I felt the blood drip from my forehead and the hands of those kind people around me, my thoughts traveled to Jesus and the crown of thorns. A few Sundays earlier while Aiding laundry the thought hit me: the halo will be removed to my head.

In a flash of a moment I saw Jesus in my mind's eye standing with the crown of thorns around His. I knew then that part of my inner spiritual work was working through my own crown of thorns inside the halo.

As you point during the Gamma Knife procedure I pressed my eyes and looking through the weight iron since upon my face there to my right stood Jesus as surely as anyone else in the room, surrounded in golden light with the crown of thorns clearly about His head.

Inwardly I looked Him. How did you do it? How did you stand it all through Your crown of thorns? wasn't alone and neither are you,

was His gentle reply.

It is a miracle that my heart started again, but it from the airplane or self-revealed.

It is a miracle that the second tumor was found and could be part of this miraculous procedure now versus showing up on an MRI six months or a year later and having to go through yet another procedure.

It is a miracle that not once did I feel alone prior to, during ever since in this journey, this time, still, now, as I continue my recovery and self-remedies.

It is a miracle that one Sunday evening in May 1997 after a long trip of home-hunting in Delaware as Kenny Ash and I were on our way to our home in Crownsville, we saw the sign "Crownsville" off 301. We knew we had to drive through just by the name itself.

We parked as we walked the town Square and as we walked the town within minutes we both knew and felt in our hearts we were home. As we crossed the street toward Mout's Barber Shop, a man stood leaning on the balcony above, in his plaid short sleeve shirt and jeans. That man said "aren't you the new folks in our new little town by our first new friend, Phil The Barber.

Since stepping public from my per-

sonal world as my last column, Jam K, so many of you in my little town have made sure I knew I was not alone. Your prayers, thoughts, hugs, cards of well wishing and calls of the same continue to fill my Grateful Heart. How could it not continue beaming? Your town is a miracle that keeps life growing and I thank you.

I shared the news of my upcoming challenge with the staff and students of Light Faith prior to the column in print.

Immediately, The Reiki Angel Team

started clearing my weekly Reiki sessions and the hours they would send healing through the hospital experience.

During the day of the procedure starting as early as 6:30 a.m. periodically as I could I would raise a thick and I knew while was with me. The calm within was matched by the smile of radiance love received and the light of radiant healing beaming in my eyes.

Thank you dear ones, thank you. Your healing work makes miracles.

Now the the Gamma Knife machine is turned off and the magic that is in Dr. Steiners M.D.,PhD. the doctor protection of Greg, Registered Nurse, the calming of Mary's, Medical Center Specialist, worth over the works, the gentle assurance of Science, Nurse Practitioner, before and after surgery, the silken presence of Lisa, Nurse Practitioner to step down ICU, and the open minded approach of Dr. Mark Quinn, Neurologist, all from the realm and kingdoms of Healing Entities energized by the University of Virginia Hospital are there and not here with our philosophy.

Yet, inside my body the miracle of restructuring my team's DNA continues on for at least the next two years and their miracle reach into my life for that lifetime and forever.

Miracles are defined as "A supernatural event or happening regarded to an act of God." (Webster's New Complete Desk Reference Book) or considerably "The use of Universal Laws beyond mortal comprehension. There is no meaning Universal Laws they are neither invisible nor alterable." (New Dictionary of Spiritual Thought by Rev. Carol Parish)

I have long ago learned that miracles surround our experiences and we need only to open our eyes, hear with our hearts and know from the very every day life and as we live and breath and know our miraculous being surrounds.

Know that I have a Grateful Heart filled with each of you as you have made miracles in my life and together as a community we live amidst All Day Everyday Miracles. Start cheering and affirming yours. It's Just A Thought, which in and of itself is a miracle.

You can learn more about the work of The Reiki Angel Team complementing your healing as well as classes, workshops and retreats held at Light Faith, Centre For The Healing Arts and The Sophia School of Wisdom by checking our Web site at www.lightfaith.org or calling 410-758-3633.

All day, every day miracles

From the Record Observer, Page A7
July 20, 2007

"Uh Oh. Quick I need an ammonia tab! I'm going, quick. I'm leaving!"

"She's back. You put a little excitement into our day. Your heart stopped."

"Ken, during the Halo MRI we found a second brain tumor." As I felt the blood drip from my forehead and the hands of those kindly wiping it away, my thoughts traveled to Jesus and the crown of thorns. A few Sunday's earlier while folding laundry the thought hit me, the halo will be screwed to my head.

In a flash of a moment, I saw Jesus in my mind's eye standing with the crown of thorns around His. I knew then what part of my inner spiritual work was working through my own crown of thorns into the halo.

At one point during the Gamma Knife procedure, I opened my eyes and looking through the wrought iron fence upon my face there to my right stood Jesus as surely as anyone else in the room, surrounded in glorious light with the crown of thorns etherically about His head.

Inwardly I asked Him, How did you do it? How did you stand at all through Your crown of thorns? "I wasn't alone and neither are you," was His reply.

It is a miracle that my heart started again, be it from the atropine or self-resolve.

It is a miracle that the second tumor was found and could be part of this miraculous procedure now versus showing up on an MRI six months or a year later and having to go through yet another procedure.

It is a miracle that not once did I feel alone prior to, during nor since in this journey, this time, still now, as I continue my recovery and self-recreation.

It is a miracle that one Sunday evening in May 1997, after a long day of house hunting in Delaware as Kenny, Asti and I were on our way to our home in Crownsville, we saw the sign "Centreville" off 301. We knew we had to drive through just by the name itself.

We parked in the Court House Square and as we walked the town within minutes, we both knew and felt in our hearts we were home. As we crossed the street toward Mear's Barber Shop, a man stood leaning on the balcony above in his plaid short-sleeve shirt and jeans. "That your dog?" were the first words spoken to us in our new little town by our first new friend, Phil the Barber.

Since stepping public from my personal world in my last column, June 8, so many of you in my little town have made sure I knew I was not alone. Your prayers, thoughts, hugs, cards of well-wishing and calls of the same continue to fill my Grateful Heart. How could it not continue beating? Your love is a miracle that keeps life growing and I thank you.

I shared the news of my upcoming challenge with the staff and students of Light Paths prior to the column in print.

Immediately, The Reiki Angel Team started charting my weekly Reiki sessions and the hours they would send healing through the hospital experience.

During the day of the procedure, starting as early as I could, I would view a clock and I knew who was with me. The calm within was matched by the smile of love received and the light of radiate healing beaming in my eyes.

Thank you, dear ones, thank you. Your healing work makes miracles.

Now the Gamma Knife machine is turned off and the magic that is Dr. Steiner, M.D., Ph.D., the all-day protection of Greg, Registered Nurse, the calming of Mary's Medical Center Specialists words over the weeks, the gentle assurance of Selene, Nurse Practitioner, before and since surgery, the silken presence of Leia, Nurse Practitioner, in step down ICU, and the open minded approach of Dr. Mark Quigg, Neurologist, all from the realms and kingdoms of Healing Entities employed by the University of Virginia Hospital are there and not here with me physically.

Yet, inside my body the miracle of restructuring my brain's DNA continues on for at least the next two years and their miracle touch into my life for this lifetime and forever.

Miracles are defined as "A supernatural event or happening regarded as an act of God." (Webster's New Complete Desk Reference Book) or esoterically "The use of Universal Laws, beyond mortal comprehension. There is no escaping Universal Laws: they are neither breakable nor alterable." (New Dictionary of Spiritual Thought by Rev. Carol Parish).

I have long ago learned that miracles surround our experiences, and we need only to open our eyes, hear with our hearts and know from the wisdom within that miracles are ordinary everyday life stuff as we live and breathe and have our miraculous being consciously.

Know that I have a Grateful Heart filled with each of you as you have made miracles in my life and together as a community, we live amidst All Day Everyday Miracles. Start claiming and affirming yours! It's Just A Thought, which in and of itself is a miracle.

Lessons to be learned — Gratitude is The Attitude

Just a Thought

Rev.
Regina
Maria
Cross

Light Pang Cross for the Healing Arts

Lessons to be learned – Gratitude is The Attitude

From the Record Observer, Page A7
November 9, 2007

I have a framed print on my office desk as well as on my vanity of a young girl looking much like Laura Ingels from Little House on the Prairie.

She is standing high on a hill. The winds are blowing her long curly red hair and the clothes she wears, a prairie dress, bloomers and gingham apron.

Her Soul's bliss is shining upon her face up to the heavens, and her arms are stretched out wide fingertip to fingertip as if embracing the world and all life has to offer.

I found this print about four years following my craniotomy on Nov. 16, 1989 (18 years ago and still blissfully counting!) and life was becoming "ordinary" again.

I could sweep, get the fork in my mouth when I aimed for it, find most words without difficulty. I could walk, and I was afraid, terribly afraid of life becoming ordinary. I was afraid I would forget my bliss. I was afraid I would forget to be grateful that I could sweep, eat without disfiguring myself, find the words and walk.

So, I cried for six months in fear forgetting to be grateful of life as it was.

One day when Kenny, my husband, came home after a long day's work, he found me crumbled on the floor in a pool of tears.

"What's wrong?" he asked. "I am so afraid I will forget all I have learned and then I will stop learning as life is becoming ordinary."

With the deep understanding of one who had been through the non-ordinary for a very long time, he looked at me and said, "Ordinary is good, really good."

It was then I understood it was up to me to remember. It was up to me to live in gratitude. It was not something that was and will no longer be because I am living an ordinary life but be because I am living an ordinary life consciously.

Gratitude is an Attitude.

Then I found this card and it was as if someone, who had seen into my Soul — claiming its innocence and sheer bliss and being able to do more than draw stick figures with really cool shoes (my forte) — created me without fear on the front of a card.

Shortly after finding this mini me in color, I found a Far Side card that to this day still gives me the giggles. On the front is a man focused on walking, really focused on walking, through his neighborhood. There are houses, picket fences, a dog, a cat, and a bird flying above him, blue skies and green grass. The caption is "I'm Walking. I'm Walking." When you open the card it says, "Ordinary is Good." Ordinary is good, really good.

Why wait to be grateful? Thanksgiving is nice. It gives us reason to get together with the whole family (really, that could be good), eat too much (most likely dysfunctionally) and do the after big dinner comatose stare.

But what if Thanksgiving were every day without the dysfunctional eating? What if we were to open our hearts to the idea that all experience is given to us, co-crafted by us if you will, for the very reason of growing us, evolving us into who God already made us to be, a Divine Spark of His/Her DNA?

It is so easy to be grateful when all is on an upswing. When you survive the prognosis of having less than a 20 percent chance of making it off the table, life is not ordinary.

But what about the ordinary day to day like being with your husband, your children, your family, friends, neighbors, doggies, kitty cats and even those you see every day but don't know by name.

Because it is ordinary, we expect it, they, will always be there. I have found that to be less than true in the last three weeks as I have as a friend and minister been involved in three memorials for three young men ages 21, 23 and 25. Suddenly they are gone and that's anything but ordinary.

How can we possibly be grateful for experiences such as these?

How can we possibly be grateful when bad things happen to good people?

Therein lays the challenge, the test if you will, of the truth of our gratitude from a spiritual perspective. "Life is wonderful even when it sucks" is one of my known saying around Light Paths.

I don't believe it, but it helps me affirm what I want to believe, what I want to know—and that is we are here to be happy, to grow as spiritual beings having an earthly experience to love one another without fear, without judgment — which is fear, so fear is the bottom line.

Oprah says, "There are only two emotions and they are love and fear. What is not love is fear and what is fear is not love." I love me, my Oprah!

So, as you approach this Thanksgiving holiday, think of the ordinary and how it is we can all bring Thanks Giving, the Giving of Thanks, into our ordinary daily routine, making Gratitude our Attitude for living an Ordinary Life.

Just a Thought…

Happy Thanks Giving every day.

Chapter Six

In Closing

"Ordinary is Good. Ordinary Is Real Good."

"Maybe one of these days I'll be able to give myself

a gold star for being ordinary,

and maybe one of these days, I'll give myself a gold star

for being extraordinary, for persisting.

And maybe one day I won't need to have a star at all."

Sue Bender

I was terrified if I healed all the way, I would not be as perfect as I am right now in my imperfection. I was afraid I would lose all the mystical guidance the Universe had gifted me through the horrendous ordeal of brain surgery and the sometimes scary, sometimes exhilarating process of creating my new normal life. I was fiercely frightened I would forget the Blessing of the Bliss while cultivating the wisdom of lessons learned challenged in life's mundane daily rounds. 'Tis the Soul's captivating reason for living a life fulfilled.

I had been realizing more and more what I could do. I could sweep without becoming dizzy. I could drive the car again. I could take my list to the store, retrieve what was necessary, lift the packages without feeling pressure in my head and drive the roads home. I could schedule my day and live it just like anyone else. Yes, I did have avenues that were new to the mapping of my life. I realized my seating placement was important anywhere if there were an overhead fan. I was aware there was memory gone forever and that remembering names was now a challenge. I knew my head hurt a lot and that I was learning more about that, the whens, wheres and whys. I knew there was a list of changes I needed to recognize and pay attention too. Yet I also knew life was becoming normal and I was frightened as never before.

What if I forgot all I had been gifted through the journey? What if I and life just became ordinary again? I would wake up and have a day and then go to bed only to wake up and have a day and then to go to bed. What if I forgot to be aware of all the new little nuances of life that I had not taken the time to be dazzled by before, like birds looking right into my eyes when they sing, centipedes and how magic it is they can use all those legs at one time to move their bodies to get somewhere, like how it is we can figure out how to do something, anything? It's all magic and what if I fall into this place of cloudy gray and nothing is as extraordinary as it truly is? What if I forget to thank Kenny every day for being here with me instead thinking, if thinking happens at all, that is the way it's supposed to be, so there it is?

I had kept this fear inside my thoughts, inside my body cavity for quite some time, maybe six months or so when suddenly one day, I strayed off course. All by myself, I thought I was safe with my secret, I collapsed falling to the living room floor in a deluge of tears I could barely breath through. I crumbled under the weight of distress thinking "it" will all be gone. "It" being all the wonder, all the Blessings, all the Bliss, all the Gratitude I felt within my Being for all I had been given through all I had been through.

There was a reason it all happened. Why a brain tumor? Why me with a brain tumor? I had yet to figure out what that reason was. Now, if I fall back into who I was, how life was, before it all began, I may never know because I won't have time in an ordinary day to place that thought in sacred space for contemplation. I won't be able to be as grateful as I could be, should be, want to be, from this place of what appears to others to be less than what I was before it all began. How am I to hold on to the wonder of ethereal bliss while living the wisdom of lessons learned challenged in life's mundane daily rounds.

Please, please, I prayed, *Don't let me forget, don't let me fall back into ordinary and forget.* I was trying to catch my breath between the waves of panicked trepidation when Kenny, coming home earlier than expected, walked into the room. His compassionate soul knelt down on the floor beside me; "What's wrong? Is your head hurting? Did you fall? What can I do? Do we need to call Kobrine?" "Kenny, I am so scared, I am so afraid...Life is becoming ordinary again....and what if...?" Kneeling in front of me, Kenny took hold of my shoulders pulling my body into an upright position. His face beaming as it would when Holy was radiating outward from his heart and soul. His smile lines shining wisdom of a life well lived. "Honey, Sweetie", his eyes now filling with tears, "You won't forget. You can't forget. Bliss is your new normal and ordinary is good. Ordinary is real good right now." His rational of the irrational continued as he explained the trek from fear to sanity in a way that abated my nightmare of forgetting the wonder. I was breathing again in rhythm to truth.

Days later while in a store as if the Universe was letting me in on the joke, I found a Gary Larson card called "Basic Lives". On the front is a man with a big toothy smile, eyes wide, walking through his neighborhood passed the trees, houses and fenced in yards. His little thought bubble says, "Left foot, right foot, left foot, right foot." The birdie flying in the sky overhead says, "Up, down, up, down, up down." The dog barking at the man walking by says, "Bark, don't bark, bark, don't bark." And the frog in the yard says, "Hop, rest, hop, rest, rest.... dang!" And he, the man, was so happy. I laughed all the way home card in hand showing Kenny my Gary card from God. Of course, he loved it laughing right along with me as the message was loud and clear. The card was blank inside until we wrote, "Life Is Good In Ordinary Times." To this day it sits framed upon my altar as a reminder just in case I do slip between the lines of gray (pun intended) momentarily forgetting, Ordinary is good. Ordinary is real good right now.

> "Ordinariness is a simple presence in this moment
> that allows the mystery of life to show itself.
> The ordinariness of spiritual life comes from
> a heart that has learned trust,
> from a gratitude for the gift of human life.
> When we are just ourselves, without pretense or artifice,
> we are at rest in the universe....
> our salvation lies in the ordinary"
>
> Jack Kornfield
> *Bringing Home the Dharma*

PART TWO

My Brain Has Taught Me These Things

Barometric Pressure
What Goes Up
Weather Call

Love The Caffeine
Bring It On

I love the caffeine only when I am in brain pain
Which is unlike any other head pain
Seriously
Love The Caffeine
With the oncoming barometric pressure changes
Be they with the storm coming or going
Love The Caffeine
When the stress pushes me to this side of overwhelm
And my head hurts
Right where the surgical site is and where the tumors are sleeping
Love The Caffeine
When my head hurts because of too much stimuli
Be it people, noise, lights, movement
You know it everyday stuff to anyone else

Research suggest drinking caffeine opens the blood vessels
Reducing inflammation
Allowing for the blood to flow freer than in the constriction of pain
Contrasting research advocates caffeine can relieve some head-brain pain
Because it blocks the ability of adenosine
(a chemical secreted by the brain)
To dilate blood vessels therefore the blood vessels constrict
When I am in brain-pain either way
Love The Caffeine
Works for me
Drinking caffeine while it does not take all the brain pain away

It does dissipate the extreme
My personal favorites 'cause they really work
Early Morning
Hot Organic Coffee with an organic flavor cream
"Pretend Coffee" as my Husband calls it
At Home During the Day
Starbucks Vanilla Frappuccino (Always keep a supply in the fridge)
On the Road
McDonald's / Starbuck's / Braum's Caramel with Hazelnut Coffee
Hot / Cold depending on weather
Something about the combination caramel and hazelnut
Loves the brain
This is my decadence and I do it for the love of my brain and me
Only when I am in brain pain
My brain taught me these things

Barometric Pressure Ball

Not a must but a good thing to have
So that you understand you are not crazy
As you can now tell the weather patterns two to four days out
By the pain you are experiencing
I could make a million being a Weather Girl
I do not need the weather ball
I've got my blessed head and brain telling me
How much rain we are going to get and where
The BP Ball allows your loved ones to understand
Why you are feeling the way you are feeling
Just like anyone else who has had broken bones
You having had your bone-head (sorry) opened
Can predict the weather
You have officially joined the Weather Girls or Guys
And it has nothing to do with T-Shirts
It really is a hoot minus the pain

A Very Wise Man Once Said

"This is when I learned much about myself and my surroundings.
In particular, I learned that, sadly, when the body becomes a prisoner of its pain
a pill or an injection is more helpful than the most brilliant philosophical idea."
*Elie Wiesel * Open Heart (Chapter 8 - Page 23)*

Or as my wise Nurse Baby Sister says "Better living through chemistry."
Sometimes a pain reliever is appropriate
Even when we do not want it to be
You have suffered enough
No need for martyrdom through recovery
Or anytime for that matter
My brain taught me these things
Check with your neurosurgeon and/or neurologist
As to what is appropriate for you

Brainium Cranium
Your Blessed Head

Bald Is Beautiful

And Brave and Bold
Bald is Awesome and Freeing and Exceptionally Cool
If you allow for the feeling to rise
There is a power unlike any other when you are a bald woman
Bald women have beaming light, truthful, bright eyes
They have intensely soulful wise eyes
You are a Warrior Woman
Bald men
Well what can I say other than hubba-hubba
Bald men are gleaming, handsome, specimens of strength
Grounded in distinctive merit
You are Super Hero Man
Bald is a badge, a statement of life's experience
The scars of surgery upon the head silently tell the story of courage
Your hair will grow back
At first kinda like baby bird butt fuzz hair
Then tiny little short nubbies
Your hair follicles reactivate
Although they may have a new understanding of to curl or not to curl
To be brown or not to be brown
Whatever
You have a head and you have your brain and until you have hair
You can get a Tina Turner, Cyndi Lauper, Katy Perry or Lady Gaga wig
Because that would be freaky fun
Dudes
If someone ask why you're wearing a scarf on your head
Tell them it's because you are a pirate
They will have no more questions
In the meantime
Bald or partial bald, scarred or not
Is Beautiful and Awesome and Powerful
Just be with it
You are not your hair

Buy A Really Cute Helmet

Protect your precious head both from the sun as well as the cold
Hats are important as are cloches and scarves
A fashion statement as well as a I Care About Me Statement
Just know that once your hair grows back
The hats you pick now as cute as they are
Are not going to fit any more
Do Not keep them - Do Not wear them
Pass them forward
You are not a clown - clowns are creepy
You are not a jester nor a fool
You are a Brilliant Brainiac
You have the scars to prove it
My brain taught me these things

Wearing Headphones

Wearing headphones under your chin
Is much better than trying to stretch them
Over your big turban brain
Or laying them over your blessed head (ouch)
Once your protective headgear is off

To calm your emotions
Your thoughts
Your heart
Your spirit
And love your brain
Listen to soothing music like Windham Hill, Jim Brickman
Or inspirational music by David Bailey who knows from whence he shares
My brain taught me these things

Freaky Hair Moments

OK
Admittedly
Hair, your hair, coming out in clumps in your hand
In the shower as you shampoo your hair
Which was attached to your head as you stepped into the shower
IS FREAKY

There is no getting around that
And it may happen
It does happen
It's gonna happen
Maybe

So be prepared
As much as one can be
For a Freaky Hair Moment
And when it does
If it does
After your first gasp of Freaky Hair Moment
Think a thought like
Well, that's different
Take a breath
A really deep breath
Exhale fully
Maybe even three deep breaths, exhaling fully
Because you may look different
Than when you last looked at yourself in the mirror

Towel off
OK, FREAKY
More hair in the towel
Breathe
Breathe some more
Cry
Really Cry
To the bottom of the last tear
For now.

And then do your very best
To be grateful you have a head

PS

There may be a morning
When you rise
Into a bright sunshiny new day
That as you turn to make the bed
You realize
Some of your hair did not follow your upward motion
Yet another Freaky Hair Moment
FHM

Nothing more you can say
It's FREAKY
As you realize
There is a breeze in the back of your head where none had been before
Gather it up gently
As it is yours
Love it
Love yourself
And as you throw it away
Flush it
Or tie it with a ribbon before you tuck it into a jewelry box
Until you decide what you will do with it
Sigh
Cry
And Smile
You have endured
Yet another very FHM
In this journey called Survivorship

MRI's

The very first MRI I ever had
I imagined the National Geographic big hooter women
Dancing in rhythm to the tribal sounds
With every magnetic beat playing through the capsule
You can enter the capsule fearful, and I have
You can enter the capsule tearful, and I have
You can enter the capsule anxious, and I have
I prefer to enter the capsule with the idea of this is my sacred space
Just for now and in this moment, this is my sacred space
Where we are about to make pretty pictures
Every time I am conveyor belted into the capsule
I remind the crew
"We are making Pretty Pictures here"
All is well because I have people out there who care about me
My Husband-Best Friend / The Techs / My Besties
My Family / and My Puppies too
Then there is my Guardian Angel and my Father-Mother God-Parents
For twenty-two years I was blessed with an MRI Trinity
In Annapolis, Maryland
Tom - Vicki - Laura
All three of them would actually change their schedule
As I made my appointment so that we could all be together
When I moved to Oklahoma that changed and I was frightened
I was lost and not someone special anymore
That is until I met Daniel at Tahlequah City Hospital
Daniel is AWESOME
He is compassionate and gentle
He even let me cry the very first time he did my MRI
Find your Tom, your Vickki, your Laura, your Daniel
Ask all the questions you need answers to
If the Techs/Docs do not answer your questions they are not your Team
You will know when you find them
The Special Them
They will take really good care of you
Once found it is a real plus if you take your team
Homemade chocolate chip cookies
And
Check it out you may notice your electrical energy field changes
Every time you get an MRI
It's just a hoot

Let's Talk Contrast

Did you really believe them when they said
"The contrast dye leaves your body
the first time you pee after your MRI"
Seriously
Wheel me out halfway through my alone time in the MRI capsule
Stick me with that big ole' needle full of yellow-orange
I don't know what goop
I can feel that sludge flowing through my veins
Like someone opened a flood gate
And it's hot
Okay warm
Just know it's possible you will feel sludge tired for a few days
Allow yourself at least three days recoup
Having been fasting prior to get yourself a really healthy meal
Then go home
Gather a good book, your pet companions, a tall glass of water
And go to bed the first day
I need daily naps for at least three days after the contrast
I also loose a palmful of hair for the next couple of shampoos
And the taste of metal (because that is what it is) in my mouth is prevalent
For a couple of weeks
A good metal detox may be in order
And if I were peeing it all out the first time I pee after my MRI
Wouldn't you think my pee may have a hint of coloring
Other than an excess of Vitamin B
Seriously

Brush, Floss, Smile, But Hold the X-Rays

Dental x-rays are a real No-No for brain tumor folks
Especially folks like me with a meningioma
Don't want to promote nor wake those babies up
Wise, compassionate dentists will instead
Take in-mouth photographs
More than likely your insurance company
Will not pay for such photographs
Even with a letter from your wise and compassionate dentist
Better to pay a small amount for mouth photos
Than deal with waking those babies up
Shhhh....Smile

Cell Phones

Okay so have you noticed that most of the studies concerning cell phones
And brain tumors have been conducted by communication companies
"Of course they don't cause brain tumors"
'Thank you very much for paying my rent and buying me a cabin cruiser'

Get yourself an EMF (Electrical Magnetic Field) Protection headset
to connect into your phone
Placing the phone as far from you as possible
Once you hook your cell phone up
It dispenses 99% of the electromagnetic radiation
That a cell phone transmits
Use your speaker again placing the phone far from your head
No foolin'
Cell phones convenient as they are
May cause the inconvenience of brain surgery
Which just may cause a major brain gap in your ability to communicate

"Of particular interest over the last decade has been the potential association between cell phone use and risk of developing a brain tumor. Multiple large studies have been performed in both the United States and Europe. Some have shown an association between cell phone use and brain tumor risk, while other studies show no association. In addition, studies have also investigated the difference in risk of a brain tumor between short-term and long-term (>10 years) cell phone use with further conflicting results. In general, the conclusions from most of these studies are (1) there is no consistent association between cell phone use and risk of developing a brain tumor (benign or malignant) and (2) there is a very slight increased risk of a brain tumor associated with using a cell phone for 10 years or more. Further studies, in both the laboratory and in humans with longer follow up, are needed to fully understand this exposure and any potential relationship with brain tumor development."

American Brain Tumor Association
*"About Brain Tumors * A Primer For Patients and Caregivers" * Page 30*

Check Out:
The Cell Tolls for Thee by Julie A. Evans
Best Life Magazine August 2008 * The Issues That Matter To Men Special Report
CBS This Morning Saturday * Bloomberg Technology * February 3, 2018
"Cell Phone Radiation Tied to Rare Tumor in Rats, Study Says"

What Was That?

A Flash
A Fire Cracker Show inside your head
Yes
Learning anew something you once just thought you knew
Like getting the fork in your mouth versus your eye
Is one thing
But
It is another thing to learn how you learn to not get the fork in your eye
Learning how your brain knows how to learn
To get the fork in your mouth versus your eye
Is even more Awesome
To feel the fire
To see the sparks
In the brain as the wheels are activated during the learning process
It's Miracle Stuff
Yes, You are feeling and seeing all that
You really can sense the wheels turning in there
And when you work on it real hard for too long
The inner brain fire really does ignite
My brain taught me these things

If You Feel / Know Something Pay Attention

If your Docs are telling you
"It's All In Your Head"
Tell them
"Yes, I know"
Pay Attention to what you feel / know
Check it out
If they still don't care
Guess what?
There are other Doctors who do
My "Pay Attentions"
When I cannot find words or do numbers
Pay Attention and Check it out
No One
No One
Knows your brain like you do
Because it's yours
No One else's

Take It In

Take in all the sensitivity to
Sight
Sound
Touch
Smell
Taste
And
Intuition
It is AWESOME
In your head
You can probably hear your blood flow through your body
At least through the beginning stages of recovery
Experience the fireworks of synapses
Your very own daily Fourth of July
As thought jumps from one end of think to the beginning of what use to be
Connected nerve endings continuing the thought process
As if finishing a sentence
It is a blessing to be this ALIVE
And to know the miracle of thinking life as you have never known it before
The extra-ordinary ability of being aware of being aware

Brain Body Olympics
Movement

Going Up Is Easy
What The Hell Happened To Going Down

Depth of Field can be confusing to the precious brain
Inside your precious head
Climbing the stairs, into the car, riding an elevator
Or for that matter climbing a tree is real easy
It's the coming down that can really confuse the brain with depth of field
As in all of a sudden there is none
Baby steps are your friend
So is holding a loved one's hand
FYI
There are two avenues of movement in the world
That just do not hold to these rules
Escalators and Airport Conveyor Walkways
Are a world unto themselves
My brain taught me these things

Head Below Heart

Sometimes it's a good thing, sometimes not such a good thing
It's a good thing when you feel an onset of dizzy, faint, or a seizure coming on
Head below Heart brings the blood flow back up into your head and brain
Bring yourself up slooooowly

Not so good a thing when you move in any direction
And it makes you dizzy
Sit down
Get down on the floor
Ground yourself and breathe slooooowly
Until you feel balanced again
But avoid staying there
People will talk

My Left Boobie Girl Hurts

Okay
So what has my left Boobie Girl got to do with Brain Surgery
You may wonder
During my first post-op visit with my most wonderful Brain Surgeon
I asked
"Doc, I know I had brain surgery so why do I have an intense straight line pain
from under my left armpit through the side of my left Boobie Girl"
Admittedly and momentarily my Doc looked a little puzzled
His eyes did that squint thing as he tilted his head up and to the right
You know the look, like someone just blew a dog whistle
As if reviewing the vista as an observer
He started to walk through the scenery out loud
"You were placed left side on the OR table
so that I could have access to right temporal lobe.
Your left arm was dangling off the side which means your left side was on the edge
Ahhh…I must have leaned a little too hard while in your brain."
So, if other than brainy parts hurt on your body after surgery
Ask so you know
No more guessing

The Righting Reflex

The innate ability to sense and correct orientation
The National Institutes of Health describes balance as
"The brain receiving, processing, and comparing visual cues
about the body's alignment
to information from our bones, muscles, joints, and ears."
Phew, what a blessed brain we have
Balance is the maintenance of one's center of gravity
While in continuous motion
Or pre/post brain surgery while sitting still
Watch a cat
You'll get there

When Simple Movement Is More Than You Can Conquer

My releasing tears
Followed by my absolute belief
Will pull me up to meet my true self again

Feed The Body
Feed The Brain
Food

Buy and Eat Only Organic

Too many toxins and pesticides can get into your beautiful brain
Pay more now, live longer and pay less in medical bills later

Keep Yogurt In The Fridge

Somehow and sometimes a good organic Greek yogurt
Alleviates brain pain
And taste good too
You might also try raw organic almonds
YUM

No Artificial Fake Sugar

Pink, yellow fake-sweet
You name it it's all really bad for your brain
Love your brain and stay far away from them all
You may be sensitive enough to feel the pain they cause
And even if you are not
They kill off short term memory cells which cannot be replaced
Say what
They can cause seizures and who needs to free fall for a diet soda
Which by the way you will not remember drinking anyway

No Wine-ing

Prior to brain surgery I could drink a gallon of Sangria
All by myself as if it were water
No effect - No problem
Not anymore
No way - No how
Now, alcohol, especially wine
Hurts my brain because it constricts the blood vessels which causes brain pain
It just hurts my whole face and really affects my vision
So drinking sucks
Don't do that
Let it go
My brain taught me these things

Don't Stand in Front of Your Microwave

Or anywhere near it
Especially with staples or a metal plate in your head
I'm just saying
Besides even without them you will most likely feel the wave
And this is one wave you do not want to catch
I push and run if I use it at all

There is a Reason They Call It Tumor-ick

Every morning I drink my special Tumor-ick drink
Today
It may be hot filtered water with a squeeze of organic lime and honey
Tomorrow
Hot organic almond or rice milk
And....Wait for it....
A teaspoon of Organic Turmeric Golden Paste
I Love It
Or take Turmeric Curcumin capsules
One capsule in the morning and one at night
Truly there is a reason they
They being the ancient and present day Ayurvedic Physicians
Call it Turmeric
Turmeric has assisted for thousands of years in keeping tumors suppressed
While keeping inflammation subdued
Check in with your Health Care Practitioner
I do believe it helps to keep my tumors quiet
Healthy and in a sleeping state of mind
Shhhhhhhh

Love The Self
Care

Auras

Pay Attention

Yes its cool to see and vibe in on yours and other's auric energy fields
Nevertheless I am talking about the pre-seizure auric energy field
That only you know
Only you see, smell, feel around you as a warning to get to your safe place
One of mine is smelling Fritos
When there is no bag of Fritos within twenty-five miles
I know kinda crazy
Yet it has been one of my clues to get to my safe place since I was a little girl
So I do pay attention to smelling Fritos when there are no Fritos around
Just in case you blow off the Frito Auric Warning or yours in particular
Now is the time to start paying attention
To your little dog paying attention to you
They know things you do not
They see, smell, feel things you may not be aware of in the moment
We learned this with our first little Yorkie, Asti Spumante
He started taking on the role of warning me about oncoming seizure activity
Now when I may not be paying close enough attention to myself
And/or the Fritos flag
Or I may have crossed over the very thin line
Into the seizure field of activity
Our sweet Yorkies Princess Cozy and Prince Dewey keep check on me
Each pup has a different warning system
And they can alert all day and all night
Through their little helpful hearts desires
Yet if I am not in tune with them I will lose the communication all together
We must be on the same page in the same intuitive breath at all times
If I am to pick up on their language of care
Cozy Cosette and Dewey Meagain have also been trained to respond
Should I have an episode

While we are on the subject of paying attention to Auric Warnings and Fritos
You may want to become aware of where you sit in public in regards to
Noise
Crowds
And
Ceiling Fans are everywhere
Ceiling fans go round and round and most people think that's it
It's not
They also go round and round in reflections
On spoons, glasses, dishes, eyewear, windows
Cell phones, jewelry, wall shadows and the list goes on just as the beat goes on
And if you want it to continue to do so without seizure interrupt-us
Be aware of choosing your seated position in public arenas
So that the movement of the reflection of ceiling fans is as safe as possible
Which makes you as safe as possible
My brain and our Yorkies taught me these things

A Button Push Away From Calm

If you are alone afraid and about to seizure
Coming out of a seizure, a panic attack, a WTFritos moment
Dial 911 First
Then
Go to people in your phone Contacts under Favorites
There is a reason they are your Favorites
You are one button push away from calm
This is not the time to hesitate, to be shy, nor ask yourself if you are worth it
Should something life changing happen
And you find yourself on the other side
Do you want to have to answer to yourself
Was the moment of repeated self-doubt worth it
Push the button
Your Favorites will be pissed if you don't
Even though calling for help means you must first blow through
I never need help I am here only to serve Sainthood Therapy
Calling gives someone else the momentarily Halo Shine
Do it for them
Yeah, yeah, that's the ticket
There ya' have it
Feel better

Be Accepting

You may be more aware of your sensitivity to
Heat
Cold
Touch
Sound
And
Emotions
Yours and others'
Be accepting and honor your needs
Be kind to you
Then again you may not be able to tell if you are cold or hot at all
So take a clue from others
If they are wearing a sweater, wear or take a sweater with you
If others are peeling off the outer wear, peel off the outer wear
Of course there is a limit to the peeling off
Don't fall for that one

Buy a Totally Captivating Bell

A charming delightful bell
As yelling for help sucks energy and hurts your head
Buy a bell so you do not have to call out for assistance when you need it
And nobody is in the same room
Buy a bell because when you try to call out to someone
You are hearing not only your outside head voice that you are used to
Now due to surgical sensitivity
You are also hearing your inside head voice that you think is louder than it is
Yet nobody else hears
So to avoid yelling which makes your head hurt and makes you want to cry
Because it is such a crackling vibration in your energy field
Buy a really cute tinker sound bell and use it

Cellular Memory

It's real
It is your bodies way of healing the past
Honor its truth
I have been through this
On this day, last week, a month, a year, a decade
Many decades ago anniversaries
I have been through this
Hello, it's me
We went through this together
Remember
I do
Me
Your Body
Honor and care for the memory
Your body holds
As it momentarily relives the experience
You may feel nearly the same pain
Physically, Emotionally, Mentally, Spiritually
It is healing itself
A magical miracle
Allowing you a moment in gratitude
For all that is now

Cognitive Reserve

Is the brain's ability to cope with injury
Our brains are 3 pounds of magical, marvelous miracles
Take good care to
Sleep well
Redirect stress
Let go of the smoke
Enjoy family and friends
Drink in moderation if at all
Enjoy brain healthy foodstuff
Exercise to your heart's delight
Soak up one new smartness everyday
Protect your precious brain from impacts and toxins

Complementary Care

If you attune to complimentary integrative infusion functional
Whatever word you are comfortable with Therapies
Go for it
No matter the judgement you may incur from others
This is your life to live as they have theirs
Remember they in their way love and care for you
Be grateful for their perception
As you remember healing is Do No Harm
Do your homework through search and discernment
I used Magnet Therapy during my recovery
Unbeknownst to all
Except Kenny my Best Friend-Husband and Pattie my Baby Sister Nurse
Ken's family Doctor, Dr. Philpott, was the top researcher at the time
(Check NIH, Magnetic Therapy and Dr. Philpott)
It did relieve my pain for 20-90 minutes at a time
That works for me 20-90 minutes at a time

Naps Are Good

Naps are good when you are tired
And do not understand why you are tired
Even though part of your head was on another table for a moment in time
While your blessed Neurosurgeon worked inside
The other half of your head and whole brain
Naps are good when you are in pain
This I did not understand or believe until my second brain surgery
I was in a great deal of brain pain one afternoon
Kenny, my Beloved, pressed me to try napping
Low and behold the man is right again
Naps do help relieve the pain
I think they just help your body and your precious brain to relax enough
Coming to the aid of your blood vessels dilating
Relaxing the constriction of pain in your brain
Napping is good for you and all those around you
My brain and my Beloved taught me these things

Nightie Night

Turn off the phone, the computer and the TV
Two to three hours before going to bed
Those tiny little lights inside each of them rob you of melatonin
Which robs you of a good night's sleep
It is a challenge in the beginning
Yet do you need to stay that connected 24/7
NO
We Do Not
What you do need to stay connected to
Is you and your precious brain and body
And the experience you are living through called your new life
I dare you to try it for a month
You will be blessed
With an enlightened understanding of bedtime preparation
And what a good night's sleep is
Nobody else can do your sleep
Which is pivotal to your present-day healing process
And your continued well-being
It's all good
Nightie Night

Pillows Are of Major Importance

Find the right pillow that allows you to actually sleep a deep sleep
It was years before I could lie down flat
And even longer before I could lay on my right side
The site of surgery
It took me years to find the pillows that allow me
To sleep a good deep restful sleep without noticing pain through the night
I found two that work best for me
A Chiropractic Water Pillow
The water pillow you fill to your preference and let water out when you want
It is soothing and cooling and it cradles my head in a soft embrace
A Bamboo Pillow
Nope seriously it looks nothing like the stalk
It has a cervical curve on both width sides, one larger than the other
I fluctuate between the two depending on my head and neck needs of the night
Ahhhhh
Nightie Night and Sweet Dreams
Check out my two favs
ChiroFlow Water-Base Pillow
Miracle Bamboo Pillow

Reiki Helps Relieve Brain Pain

Kenny would put his big man hands on my surgical site
With his purest intention
"I want Regina out of pain"
That's all
He never once said "I will take on her pain"
He just wanted to relieve his Beloved of pain
I could feel the pain being drawn out and dissipating through his hand
Never once was he caught up in it
We did not know until 5 years later that it is called Reiki
Hands on Healing through Universal Life Force Energy
Universal Life Force Energy for me is The Essence of God
We knew it worked having come in through the back door
We were trained in The Usui System of Traditional Reiki Healing
It works, really works
Try it
You will like it
Reiki has no ties to doctrine nor religion
Many Spiritual affiliations have a Hands On Healing Technique
Seek and Ye Shall Find
My brain taught me these things without me knowing

Reward Attention

When dog food kibble shakes off the serving spoon
When your lipstick case slips from your hand for no good reason
When you think the word "possible" and say "forever"
When you can't find the words or do the numbers
When the "o" is an "i" on your iPhone
Brain things are happening to get your attention
Reward attention
It's probably nothing
And
You know who you are
And how your brain works better than anyone
Go see your Doctor, Therapist, Health Practitioner
Reward attention and breathe easier

Trying To Find Words

When people are being kind, trying to find words to make you feel better
They may say things you do not need to hear
Place your fingers to your lips smile and say
"Shhhhhhhh"
"I need to grieve / heal in my own way"

Who You Are

Never make yourself
Your Experience
An excuse
For being less than who you are

Sentiments of the Heart
Emotions

Anger
Frustration
All Round Pissy
You Have The Power Of Choice

Anger hurts your head your brain
There may be times when you feel so frustrated
That you build it into a moment of anger
Remember that anger is only the front face of pain
Be it sadness, grief, or physical
Better to deal with the sadness of your perspective
Of what is in the moment
Your grief of what is no longer can be replaced with your new authentic self
The actual physical "brain pain" you are feeling is real
You have the power of choice
Be kind to you

Crying Hurts

It does but sometimes less than not crying
Give yourself permission to feel all that you are feeling
Sadness
Grief
Guilt
Bliss
Love
Joy
Yes, Awesome makes you want to cry too
Then go take a nap

When Others Get Upset About Your Memory Loss

Allow them their sorrow without you taking it in or on
Their perspective is from where they are
Not from where you live nor have lived
Now will live, with or without the memory including this, their moment
If and when you misplace a memory embroider a new one
Right here
Right now

Honor The Day

Every year Kenny Celebrates with Me
October 19
The Day of Diagnosis 1989 and The Day of my Ministerial Ordination 2003
November 16
The Day of My Craniotomy Surgery * My Brain's Second Birthday
June 26
The Day of My Gamma Knife Procedure * My Brain's Other Birthday
Maybe a special drive away to a place we've never been and dinner
Whatever I plan
We plan
I / We want to Celebrate Miracles

The Day of Diagnosis
The Day of Surgery
The Day you went Home
In whatever way you want to honor you and your journey
Prayer - Meditation - Talk - Buy me something
Go out to a special meal
Write a letter
To Yourself
To Your Brain
Loved One's who saw you through
Your NeuroSurgeon
The Hospital Staff
(Believe me that's something that rarely happens for them)
Watch a Special Inner Soul Connection movie
Again
"Phenomenon"
"50 First Dates"
"Heart and Souls"
A few of my favorites

Or if ignoring
Forgetting is your honor of self and the event
"Forget about it"
But you know you won't
Because you are remembering to ignore it
Aren't you lucky?

Seriously
Who Would Have Thought

Accept It
It's Gonna Happen

Someone opened a door in your brain and forgot to shut it
Before the surgery was over
You just may say things as you are waking from anesthesia
Crazy wild where did that come from things
Things that forever people are going to remind you came out of your mouth
Who would have thought those words would come out of my sweet
Raised a Good Catholic Girl
Your affiliation/denomination here _____
Never did anything outside the box, mouth
And there will be witnesses
Witnesses you cannot attest to their presence being a reality
Because you were still under a major drug induced brain fog
This could just be one of the most embarrassing moments in your life
You just won't know to be shamed, mortified or even chagrined
Nor will you remember the moment at any time during your life
As those who were there repeatedly and sporadically remind you
Of its absolute truth

Okay, here it is
My Witnesses
Kenny my Best Friend-Husband
Pattie-Poo my Baby Sister the Nurse who knows things
And yes The Recovery Room Nurse
The first words out of my mouth as I started my new life
Waking from a 6+ hour brain surgery
A brain surgery I had less than a 20% survival
A brain surgery that if I did survive, I had an 80% possibility
Of being in a vegetative state
They say I opened my eyes, looked at Kenny and said
Wait for it....
"Climb on up here Big Boy and do me!"
Holy Crap
What part of my brain did that come from
NEVER...NEVER....NEVER
Had I ever said anything like that before in my wakeful conscious life
NEVER

I fell back into recovery sleep only to briefly wake 20 minutes later
This time crying desperately as Kenny held my hand
"Honey we won't be able to do it for a really long time.
I just had brain surgery."
Say WHAT
Then fast drug induced sleep for a long, long time
Nope
As Kenny, Mom and Pattie came in to kiss me recovery room good-night
I heard Mom say "Her Father is waiting out in the car and we should go"
My out loud of my mouth response
"I just had brain surgery
You tell Dad to get his butt in here and kiss me goodnight"
Seriously never spoke like that to my Dad or anybody
EVER
But he did and with a smile on his face I heard him say "Nightie Night"
Accept it's gonna happen
And you will never live it down
Kenny and Pattie taught my brain these things

Make It Up and Have Fun While You Do

Who
Say What
That is too a word
Seriously, the name file went with the first brain tumor
Right along with high school and a boat load of family memories
So play games to remember a name
In Wonderland...Alice
She's daffy...Daisy
Your mustache reminds me of my uncle...Charlie
Lots of folks forget names and they didn't have brain surgery
What's their excuse
Words are a funny thing
Who made them up anyway
Creative Thinkers
Brain Tumor Survivors
Creative Brain Tumor Survivor Thinkers
Kenny is always saying I should write my own dictionary
I still think Understandment should be a word
Commitment is
Enlargement is
De-Scare makes sense to me and I know what I mean when I use it
Mush-Brain means *I'm Done Must Stop Can Think No More*
That works
Wonderment
Is that a purely wonderful word or what
Totally captures it all
Kenny still lets me know when he is going outside
To vacuum and cool-whip the lawn
And I appreciate knowing what he is talking about
And I really appreciate that he knew what I was talking about when I said it

Seriously
Who Made Up Numbers

Really
Who decided One = 1
Two = 2
And so forth or is that Fourth
Who made that up

Sky Diving

Don't
And if you are still tempted
Make sure you check with your Neurosurgeon before you do
After a long perplexing silence over the phone, mine just said
"No, You can't do that. You can't even go up in the plane"
Something to do with the cabin pressure or lack thereof
I was okay with that as it got me an answer from my neurosurgeon
That got me out of having to say No only from scaredy-cat me
Phew
Like who's gonna question your Neurosurgeon

The Aha Moments
Be In Them

Be with them
The Aha Moments of "I know this"
They are that millisecond of life when you realize
I knew that — Now I really know this
Embrace them
Bathe in them
Marvel at them
Take pure pleasure in their appearance
Be surprised and shaken by your current wisdom
Know that you have illuminated yet another new spark
In your brilliant brain
Where memory of this one
Until the next one
Resides in a forever and ever awesome you
Amen

Spiritual
The Mystical Intangible

Create Your Self Nurturing Rituals

Waking to a New Day
You get another
Going to bed
Ahhh - Rest
Loving and Accepting You Now
No apologies
After all
What are you apologizing for

"Stressed Souls need the reassuring rhythm of self-nurturing rituals"
So says Sarah Ban Breathnach in her Self-Nurturing
Book *"Simple Abundance A Daybook of Comfort and Joy"*

Death and Dying

This too in a sense you have already done
Be honest
After hearing your diagnosis
What was your second thought once you collected yourself
It may have been the truth
A high percentage possibility of your death through this journey
It becomes a way of thinking, living and planning
If not admittedly subliminally for sure
Now you have survived
You have more than survived
You are soul thriving
Having been there
Death and Dying
And back
There is no need now to fear what is true for every living sentient being
Life behind the Door of Death
Live Well
Die Well

Grieve

Who you were before diagnosis
Grieve
What has become a dearly precious time of deep soulful caring in your life
Ask
Will tomorrow be normal
Ordinary
What does that mean
After your New Life since diagnosis
And living through the healing
Now is the time to create the New Ordinary
Rejoice in your Rebirth

Hug Freely

Hug your Surgeon
Hug your Nurse
Hug your Caretakers
Often
Because you can
And they generally don't know how
Because they have been taught
Self or otherwise
Not to do so as to distance themselves from attachment
To you
Your outcome
You and/or their emotions
Seriously how's that working for ya'
With your hug teach them you are bonded
Show them your gratitude
With arms outstretched wide
Warn them
Big Hug Comin' Atcha'

I Am Careful About My Language

For so long there was so much I could not do
I am careful when using words like
Not
Can't
Don't
Forgot
I use them only in dire times of emphasis
Instead I use
I Am
I Accept
I Choose
I Remember
Your brain is listening
It believes you and it does as you tell it
We are here to En-Lighten-Up
Our brain is one vehicle allowing us to do so
And our mind flows
My brain taught me these things

I Love My Brain and My Mind

My mind housed in my brain has the ability to choose thoughts
Thoughts that create my present as well as my future
I choose thoughts that are positive, creative, calm, and delightful
I choose to breathe fully through life's pleasantries as well as its challenges

It's Simple

Every morning you wake
Open your eyes
And
Give Thanks
"For waking me This Side of Life"

Join The Brain Buddy Club
Or Start Your Own

We are a rare find
When survivors meet
A momentary flicker passes between the eyes
As if to say
I know I've been there and just as I did you will come out the other side
We have our own celebrated language
When you speak it to another who knows
There is be no need for translation
You who are in the beginning mist of the journey
Become a saving force because of who you are
And your heart smiles

Keep Each and Every Card

They are full of wishes and prayers
For your strength through the challenges and recovery from the trauma
Keep them for years and decades
Read then now and again
Reminding yourself how dearly and deeply
You are loved by so many

Leave The Analysis to the Analyst

We are all born with God Gifts
Should yours heighten through this journey
Leave the analysis to the analyst
Abandon the scrutiny
Questioning your endowment
The Giver just may take it back behind the Veil
In thought you are not ready for it
Smile, learn, accept it or them and show gratitude
My brain and my soul taught me these things

Meditate
Be Alone
Take Pleasure in Solitude

"Put your ear down next to your Soul and listen hard"
Advises the poet Anne Sexton
Center your thoughts
Calm your emotions
Align your Being
Breathe in Love
Only Love
Feel Joy
Be Joy

Share

Share and Share and Share Some More
Your Heart
Your Story
Your Authenticity
You have no idea who you will touch this day
Making a possible slight difference
An easy change
A gentle modification in their thought, word and deed
From where they are to where they want to be
Because of who you are
You have graduated from patient to physician of the soul
The experience you have lived through
And the life you are authentically living
Matters

Write Your Own Life Story

There were times I could not write
Too weak
Too deep
Lacking the vocabulary for what it was
Yet the language of the exact words in the moment are most important
It is a new self-conversation
You are a mystic wordsmith gifted with a blank sheet of paper
An artist of life with a fresh palate of oils
Record your written words as the voice writes for you
Write for your self

Remember, It's All Spiritual
Souls, including your own, are eternally alive.

The Be-Attitudes

Be a Possibilitarian

Remember
Positivity can be as simple as
Deciding what to wear
Tomorrow
Because tomorrow will come
And you will be here to greet the day

Believe in Your New Authentic Self

Keep your newfound innocence
Guard it with your breath
As if romancing your Soul Mate
Never
Ever
Let another kill your Spirit

Be Grateful

Always and forever
Be grateful for the Bigs and the smalls
Sometimes the smalls are the Bigs

Be Prepared

At least in thought for those who were prepared you would die
They may leave your life
For now or forever
Let them go
Your grief will come
Be gentle with yourself
Take from them what you will
Breathe life into your lessons learned
Know you are not responsible for their journey
Through your life

Did You Know That You Can Part The Clouds?

"I've looked at clouds from Both Sides Now
From up and down and still somehow
It's clouds illusions I recall
I really don't know clouds at all"
Judy Collins was right
But you can
Know them that is
Truly you can
Laughingly in total communication they let you

Kenny taught me how in the Spring following my first Brain Surgery
We were told "20 minutes up, 20 minutes down"
When down I was to be in a seated upright position
So my Best Boy-Friend created for me
My very own special Bedroom Tree Bench
Under our very special Bedroom Tree
The one we could see outside the window from our bed
My very own Outside Caring Room in the shade
He sat with me and showed me how to part the clouds
How to play with them
Dance with them
Laugh with them
In asking them to do what I wanted to see them do
Low and behold
They did
Move to the left... Move to the right... Move up... Move down... Make a donut hole
Check it out
Play Play Play
And never forget the miracle playmate they are
Okay try to never forget

Do Your Best

To Be Your Best
And somedays
Everyday
You will get there

Find Your Own Survival Tunes

Songs
Tunes
Words
Music
Melodies
Are healing gifts from the universe
Yours are not another's
Any more than another's is yours

I tried sharing
No one connected to mine like me
"That's nice" they would say
Nice
That tune, those words rescued me
Every time I listen to "Regina's Brain Music"
I travel heart and soul to the cellular memory of blissful gratitude
As all distractions disappear my mind, body, emotions, and soul
Refocus on the reality of what is truly important and why I am still here
The very fact that I am still here
My brain taught me these things

Gathering Information

Don't make up stories
Before you get there
Before you know
It's easy to do
Being in your head
What was your first thought when you heard
Brain Tumor
Death and dying, right
Wrong and not always
Being in your head is easy to do
Be in your calm
Making up stories is worrisome
Wait until you know the truth
Then think
Then act
Then be

Hire Yourself an Alternative Thinker

Okay, eventually you will have to send them hiking
Or better as I did place them on retainer
My sweet Kenny and my sister Terry were my alternative thinkers
Pick one
Maybe two
Designated Alternative Thinking Drivers of Thought
There may be another way out of the bag
Being stuck in only one way of thinking
Is just that
A One Way Road
There are alternatives
And your brain just hasn't found the detour highway just yet
No need for frustration
Instead celebrate you and your alternative thinkers
Ask them often
"What part of your brain did that come from"
When the time comes
And it will come
Your own reserve auxiliary files open up
When you have thought of more than one way of doing
Resolving
Opening the bottle
Keep those brilliant twinkle eyed people on retainer
You have been boosting their brain waves
Keeping them employed through your healing process
The brain is a most marvelous playground
Stomp
Dance
Run
Through your brain's nature reserve

I Am Very Clear

There is so little that is important in life
To that which is
Pay attention

If You Are So Inclined

Find out everything you can about Your Brain Part
My brain part was a Right Temporal Lobe Meningioma
My first tumor was so large (How large was it)
It took up residence within the neighborhood of Occipital and Parietal as well
This tumor
I.E. experience
Is part of who you are
A BIG Part
Physically
Emotionally
Mentally
And
Spiritually
Otherwise all this would not have happened as it has
Nor would you have survived it
To explore it
Should you so choose to do so
No matter the choice
Honor You
and
Who You Are
You are the only You ever created
You have Co-chosen
Co-created living Your life
Honor Your Journey

Multi-Tasking
What's Up With That?

Nobody's brain wants to
So Don't
Make the choice
Multi-Tasking
It ain't all it's cracked up to be
Honor your pace
Your perfect imperfection
And your achievements
As yours
Only Sweetly
Intimately
Uniquely Yours

And when others screw up 'cause they lost their focus
Or because they just pretend or fall into someone else's pressure to impress
Smile and know through your clear choice
And it is a choice
Your One Task At A Time
(OTAAT)
Is complete
Joyfully
Simply
Entirely

Multi-Tasking
The brain does not like it
Nobody's brain likes it

"The research is unanimous, which is very rare in social sciences, and it says that people who chronically multitask show an enormous range of deficits. They're basically terrible at all sorts of cognitive task. Including multitasking."

Clifford Nass, Professor of Communications
Stafford University
The Man Who Lied to His Laptop

No Apologies

You are fine
You are perfect
There is nothing wrong with you
You had brain surgery
This does not define you
It makes you more of who you are

No Worries

Unless there is reason to do so
And even then
No worry
Instead
Moving forward
With bright, mindful decisions
Remember the importance of language
It is as simple as changing the word from worry to concern
Listen and feel the energy
I am worried about
I am concerned about
Softer, gentler (Is that a word)
Easier to hear yourself say and be
No need to worry
No need to be concerned
About having enough strength and energy for tomorrow
Tomorrow will come with its own renewed supply
When faced with all else, repeat after me
"It ain't brain surgery"
My brain has taught me these things

Ordinary Is Good
Really Good

When your life begins to reacclimatize (Is that a word - It is Now)
Itself into your New Normal
When you can sweep
And blink
And remember more than 2 numbers at a time again
Remember
As scary as it is
Ordinary is Good
Really Good
Right where you are is perfect
In the everyday Ordinary
You are living a post enlightenment life
And Yes you will remember the lessons you gathered through this experience
It is up to you if you are going to keep them active in your life
I'm Walking
I'm Walking
I'm Walking
Walking is Good
And Wonderful
And Ordinary

Relish Your Slow Life

As pace will pick up again
Relish your slow life
Right now
Drink in all the subtleties
The raindrops
The awesome mechanics of a walk
How your leg picks itself up through your hip
The thigh
The bend of your knee
The stretch of your shin
The solid planting of your foot on the ground
All in a moment usually unnoticed
It is Miracle Stuff
Feel Your Inner Miracle Stuff A'Foot

Statistics Are An Unfinished Sentence

Remember that
"Patients in your position have a less than a 20% chance
Of living through the surgery."
"People with your type of tumor have an 80% chance of dying on the table"
"If you live you have an 80% chance of being in a vegetative state
for the rest of your life"
Well thank you for sharing
The rest of the sentence goes something like
I have an 20% chance of making it off the surgical table intact
I have a 20% chance of living a vital, awesomely healthy time on earth
for the rest of my life
Somebody has to be the 1% of the unfinished sentence
Pick Me

Statistics are essential information as a springboard for your personal
Be-Attitude
Keep in mind they apply to the general population
Accept them as that
And
I'll take it from here

Then there's
"I'm sorry there is nothing more I can do"
And you say "Okay, thank you"
Because whoever they are they are telling you the truth
There is nothing more THEY can do
That does not mean there is nothing more that can be done
And the Search begins
Again
(See Resources)

Watch Inspirational Uplifting Enlightening Movies

"Phenomenon"
"50 First Dates"
"Heart and Souls"
"Collateral Beauty"
You may recognize yourself in the characters
And if not, you will realize how lucky you are to have it so easy

You Are Not The Only One
Who Has Been Through Your Brain Surgery

There have been times when I thought
I am not sure which is worse being the person who had the brain surgery
or being the person who loves the person who had brain surgery
Kenny answered that for me once
When he overheard me sharing that thought with a client
His affirmatively loud response was
"Oh No Sucks to be You. Way worse to be You."
Your Beloveds have been traveling the roads with you
You are gifted with communication that needs no speaking
They look at your forehead and know on a rating scale of 1-10
How you are feeling and with compassionate care respond
You glimpse deeper into each other's hearts
Aware of a love neither of you knew existed
Hold tight and know you are loved
Be gentle with yourself and them as much as possible
My brain taught me these things

You Are A Survivor

Walk
Pray
Live Life
Ask for help
And
Breathe each moment as if it is your first

A Prayer For Brain Tumor Survivors

My name is Rev. Regina Maria Bernadette Cross.
On November 16, 1989, I had brain surgery.
I am honored and full of gratitude to be here today.
The following is a prayer of honor and gratitude touching into all levels of survivorship: the Physical, Emotional, Mental and Spiritual.
If you like, allow this to be a time of meditation, becoming comfortable in your place, closing your eyes, permitting your breath to ride rhythmically through your body.

Survivorship Has Many Stages:

Having a brain tumor and not knowing it, we are surviving.

Being diagnosed we become patients and we begin our survivorship journey.

Having surgery, chemotherapy, radiation, radio-surgery and other treatments, we are patients and we are surviving.

Pursuing nutrition, complimentary medicine, and wellness activities, we are survivors.

Receiving, watching and waiting, scan after scan, we are surviving.

Trying to return to what we knew as normal, we are surviving.

Realizing that life with a brain tumor causes our definition of normal to change, we are surviving.

Living with a brain tumor that may ultimately overcome this body, we survive as long as humanly possible.

We are always a survivor at the different stages of our journey.

We acknowledge and celebrate the grace, strength and vital energy of every person touched by a brain tumor.

We can pray for ourselves and others are welcome to offer their prayers for us. We can pray for each other and there is the silence of prayers never spoken by those unable to pray. We need only to be open and accepting of these prayers to benefit from their blessing.

And We Pray:

May brain tumor survivors be at ease with themselves. May we allow our anger, our tears, our grief, and our unexplained emotions along with our laughter, our bravery and our bliss.

May we be at ease with each other, allowing the same.

May those who are struggling with the everyday life of living with a brain tumor find comfort and strength in themselves, each other, their caregivers and their Higher Source.

May we dream courageously, act faithfully and share our inspiration as our dreams manifest.

Where there is life, there is hope.
Where there is hope, there is life.
May we be hopeful.

May we have courage to conquer our brain tumors with our words, understanding that form follows thought.

Many survivors experience their brain tumors as a gift. It grants us the truth and crystallizes the knowledge of what is truly important in life. We learn there is so little that is truly important in life. And that, so little is precious. May we always remember to treasure that which is.

May we recognize and accept the changes in us and love ourselves all the while.

If our body and face have literally been changed by the brain tumor surgery or treatment may everyone around us, including ourselves, see our Spirit and not only our flesh.

When we are tired, when we forget, when we have difficulty understanding, when we can't get it off the black-board in our mind to spell it through the pen in our hand, when we can't see as others do, when we stumble making our step a little less graceful than a dance, may we, our families and friends and those we come in contact with each day love us and accept us unconditionally.

May the stigma experienced by people with brain tumors be eliminated and so that it will be, may we be the ones to teach the truth by the way we live our life.

Grant us help in adjusting to our new normal and the understanding of the power that we have as survivors.

May others begin to understand, accept, respect and accommodate our new normal of life and power.

When we become frustrated with others' remarks that we look so good there couldn't possibly be any problems, may we give them thanks that we do look that good and then help them to understand the limit of their vision.

Let no one say that one person's brain tumor experience is more difficult than any other. It is not a contest. We are each living our own Spiritual journey enhanced by the Light together on different Paths.

May those who experience depression reach out when they can and may we reach in when they cannot.

May our prayers enhance our immune systems that we can overcome what is harmful to us.

May we have the courage to ask for help when we need it.

We give thanks for our strong support network of families, friends, employers and fellow workers.

We pray to live in harmony our Spiritual beliefs beyond faith into knowing and that it is our positive attitudes that create our membership into survivorship.

May we be free from Physical, Emotional, Mental and Spiritual pain, be it in the form of hair loss, scars, seizures, sensory loss or the look on another's face when you can't remember their name.

May our abilities be supported, not doubted.

May those who have been financially devastated by a brain tumor receive aid.

May survivors never be exploited.

May those survivors who experience survivor guilt be released from their self-torture, living a life of grace that they represent possibilities.

May they share their gifts and gained wisdom as the fortune to be given to others.

May our lay and professional caregivers be blessed with compassionate love while they share our journey with grace, finding the support they need both in others and us.

May we share with each other our strength, courage, inspiration and gratitude.

We give mighty thanks for our medical caregivers, the network of support offered and the organizations that support our new life.

May our treating physicians be hopeful.

May our health be bountiful.

If the time comes for us to make a change of worlds, may our families, friends and caregivers let us go.

May the longtime sun shine upon us.

May all love surround us and all pure Light within us guide our way on.

We pray for legislators, researchers, policy makers and business people that they have wisdom and clarity to act in our best interest.

We call upon all of the positive energy available to us in the Universes to act upon us for the good of all concerned.

May we have courage to know ourselves, sharing support with one another in our global community.

Each of us here is a gift. We are gifts to each other. It is this gift of loving that we share that sees us through.

It is the Power, the Light and the Love that restores the courage, the strength and truth of who we are.

I would like to end this prayer with a prayer I say each morning after my meditation which guides me into the perspective of the day:

"Oh Sphere of Light
Advancing and elevating Goodness
May my soul rise with You
Expressing goodness in all its contacts."

(A Daily Discipline of Worship by Torkom Saraydarian)

That is why we survive. Let us live to thrive.

Amen

May is Brain Tumor Awareness Month
Brain Tumor Action Week May 2004
Capital Hill Washington, DC
Rev. Regina Maria Bernadette Cross, Officiating Chaplain

RESOURCES

American Brain Tumor Association * ABTA
"Providing and pursuing answers."
"The American Brain Tumor Association was the first
and is now the only National Organization committed
to funding Brain Tumor Research and providing support
and education programs for all tumor types and all age groups."

Grand and Wonderful People
who will spend all the time you need on the phone with you
or your loved one.
They will send you a myriad of information
that may be of assistance to you
as you travel this unwritten road.
They have webinars, pamphlets, books, and phone numbers.
They help you, guide you and encourage you and your caregivers
from diagnosis through treatment and beyond.
They help you and your caregivers learn more of your New Me.
800-886-2282
info@abta.org
8550 West Bryn Mawr Avenue, Suite 550
Chicago, IL 60631

American Vitiligo Research Foundation, Inc.
"The American Vitiligo Research Foundation, Inc. (AVRF)
provides public awareness about vitiligo
through dedicated work, education, and counseling."
727-461-3899
www.avrf.org
vitiligo@avrf.org
P.O. Box 7540 Clearwater, Florida 33758

I add this resource because
one of the possible side effects
of the seizure medication Tegratol XR is vitiligo.
Guess who? Now I'm a painted pony in human form.
Who cares, I'm alive!
People looking at you care.
One of my sisters thought I was dying of some horrible skin cootie.
Education is key for the painted pony as well as those who love them.

AARP
A section of the aarp.org website
features the latest news and research on brain health.

Chaplains on Hand
"Offers 24/7 spiritual comfort and support to anyone,
regardless of religious beliefs."
844-242-7524
chaplainsonhand.org

National Brain Tumor Society
"We are committed to improving the lives
of all those affected by brain tumors."
617-924-9997
braintumor.org
55 Chapel Street, Suite 200
Newton, Massachusetts 02458

National Institute of Mental Health
"U.S. government institute devoted to
the understanding and treatment of illness."
www.mimh.nih.gov

National Institute of Neurological Disorders and Strokes
"U.S. government organizations that conduct and support
research on the more than 600 disorders that can affect
the brain and nervous system."
www.ninds.nih.gov

Oklahoma Brain Tumor Foundation
"The OKBTF is dedicated to serving
children, adults and their families
battling a brain tumor in Oklahoma."
405-843-4673
5235 N Lincoln Blvd
Oklahoma City, Oklahoma 73105

Society for Neuroscience
"Nonprofit organization of scientists and physicians
who study the brain.
Website features neuroscience publications
created for the general public."
www.sfn.org

The Anita Kaufman Foundation
"Anyone With A Brain Can Have A Seizure."
201-655-0420
akfus.org

The Epilepsy Foundation
"Dare To Defy Seizures"
"Our Epilepsy Resource Center Staff can answer your questions
about epilepsy, seizures, treatment, and related issues."
800-332-1000
epilepsy.com
ContactUs@efa.org
8301 Professional Place East, Suite 200
Landover, Maryland 20785-2353
P.O. Box 11
New Milford, New Jersey 07646

The Healing Exchange Brain Trust
"We host a diverse collection of online support groups"
"Group communication is by a private email list hosted by
T.H.E. BRAIN TRUST
A 501(c)(3) nonprofit organization
specializing in internet based and patient oriented
brain tumor support groups."
braintrust.org

Resources For Caregivers Well-Being
www.caringinfo.org
www.assets.aarp.org
www.womenshealth.gov
www.familycaregiver.org
www.caregiverstress.com
www.mayoclinic.com/health/caregiver-stress
www.webmd.com/balance/stress-management

Be Your Own Card-Carrying Advocate
Carry an Emergency Alert Card in your wallet
Hopefully you will never need it
And if you do, yahoo, it is there
Front side is about you
Back side about those who care
There is a page of them in the back of the book
For your card carrying convenience

While You Are At It
Carry a copy of all drug allergies
Always a hard copy and if you like in a phone App
Should something happen
Should you not be conscious
It is rather important that those who are trying to be helpful
Know not to give you a drug that could do harm
rather than be of assistance

Brain Books I Love

Dictionary for Brain Tumor Patients
ABTA
"Sharing knowledge, Sharing hope"
Truly a God Send

Living with a Brain Tumor
A Guide for Brain Tumor Patients
ABTA
Helps to calm the fears

Proof of Heaven
Eben Alexander, M.D.
"A Neurosurgeon's Journey into the Afterlife"
I rejoice in Eben's truth and his bravery (courage) for sharing it.

My Stroke of Insight
Jill Bolte Taylor, Ph.D.
"A Brain Scientist's Personal Journey"
I just want to sit with this woman and thank her immensely
for her acknowledgement of how it is.

The Human Brain Book
Rita Carter
"An Illustrated Guide To Its Structure, Function, and Disorders"

Keep Your Brain Alive
Lawrence C. Katz, Ph.D. & Manning Rubin
"83 Neurobic Exercise to Help Prevent Memory Loss
and Increase Mental Fitness"
Good fun while creating new and different patterns
of neuron activity in your brain!
Expect to clean the bathroom mirror
after brushing your teeth with your non-dominate hand.
Hehehehehehe

The Wonder of The Brain
Gopi Krishna
"By a strange dispensation of Providence,
the author of this book was led to an internal observation
of his own brain..."
Often while reading this book my breathing pattern changed
while understanding from whence he writes.

Gray Matter
David Levy, MD with Joel Kilpatrick
"A neurosurgeon discovers the power of prayer...
one patient at a time."
Thank you, David, for your courage to say so
in a field where many are taught
if you can't graph it, it does not exist.

Where God Lives
Melvin Morse, M.D. with Paul Perry
"The Science of The Paranormal
and How Our Brains Are Linked To The Universe"
Thank You, Dr. Morse, for speaking the truth of what is.

Why God Won't Go Away
Brain Science and the Biology of Belief
Andrew Newberg, M.D. & Eugene d'Aquili
"Newborn and d'Aquili show that the religions impulse
is rooted in the biology of the brain,
but is religion merely a product of biology
or has the human brain been mysteriously endowed
with the unique capacity to reach and know God?"
Magnificent!

Biology of Transcendence
Joseph Chilton Pearce
"This latest research identifies our five neural centers, or brains,
and establishes that our fourth and most recently developed brain
is located in the head while the fifth is located in the heart."
You can't help but smile.

Happy Healthy Handbook for your Brain
Prevention Hearst Specials
"Healthy Brain, Healthy Body * Challenge Your Mind
Give It A Rest * Eat For Your Memory"
A fun book of Brain Boosters on so many levels.

Navigating Through A Strange Land
Edited by Tricia Ann Roloff
"The personal stories of patients, families, and health care providers.
Resources for treatment, recovery and support."
My heart connected with so many of the folks
navigating their unchartered journey.

Brain Books I Like

How The Brain Works
Understanding Brain Functions, Thought, and Personality
General Editor: Professor Peter Abrahams
"Whether looking to identify a medical complaint,
seeking further information about a diagnosis,
or just keen to understand the processes of the human mind,
How The Brain Works is an excellent, accessible reference work
written by medical professionals."

Using Your Brain For A Change
Richard Bandler
"This book opens a doorway to a practical new way of
understanding how your mind works.
More important, this book teaches specific simple principles
that you can use to run your own brain."
I enjoyed some of this book gifting other thought than the usual
and then some of it was just too complicated
in its simplicity and a little bit mean.
Still for the other thought than the usual it was worth the read.

I had brain surgery, what's your excuse?
An illustrated memoir by Suzy Becker
Awesome genuine sharing of her experience
with heart and an irreverent wit.
And she is a sweet person in person.

Train Your Mind Change Your Mind
Sharon Begley
"A Groundbreaking Collaboration
Between Neuroscience and Buddhism"

The Plastic Mind
"New Science Reveals Our Extraordinary Potential
To Transform Ourselves"
Same book with a new title and an easier read.
Fascinating read about the miracle
of our precious brain's neuroplasticity.

Whole Brain Living
the ANATOMY *of* CHOICE *and the* FOUR CHARATERS
THAT DRIVE OUR LIFE
Jill Bolte Taylor, Ph.D.
Such fun knowing more about ourselves
and how to honor the brilliance of our brains.

Brains That Work a Little Bit Differently
Allen D. Bragdon & David Gamon, Ph.D.
"Recent Discoveries About Common Brain Diversities"
I especially related to the chapters:
"Deja Vu"
Although I do not agree with all being said it's a reality.
"Dyslexia"
I am amazed to recognize years of learning difficulties
prior to my craniotomy.
"Synesthesia"
I relate to the connections.

Evolve Your Brain
Joe Dispenza, D.C.
"The Science of Changing Your Mind'
Explore how the brain learns, processes information
and the possibility of stimulating new experiences.

Brain Games
Consultant: Elkhonon Goldberg, Ph.D.
"Lower Your Brain Age in Minutes a Day"
I didn't think I could do it. I hesitated because I didn't want to fail.
I changed the "f word" from fear to fun.
I challenged myself and was joyfully surprised again
just how awesome my brain is!
Or try
The Brain Power Workout
by Joel Levy
"300 ways to improve your memory and creativity"
Brain Boot Camp
Dr. Douglas J. Mason
"The Memory Doctor"
"Work Out Your Mind And Boost Brainpower
With Your Very Own Electronic Coach
Brain Games Kids
Publications International. Ltd.
"Power Up Your Brain!"
And/Or
Get yourself a yearly desk calendar like
Daily Brain Games by Happy Neuron

Plant a Geranium in your Cranium
Barbara Johnson
"Sprouting Seeds of Joy in the Manure of Life"
An inspiration in the medicine of laughter

Brain States
Tom Kenyon, M.A.
"...learning how to access one's deeper consciousness.
And that is why I wrote this book."

The Science Of Mind
Kenneth A. Klivington
"The purpose of this book is to help resolve dilemmas such as these:
to clarify the kinds of sensible questions that can be asked
about the function of the brain....
Intelligence, love and hate, the daily rhythms of the body,
sleep and dreams, schizophrenia and drug addiction
are all linked to the functions of the brain. But how?"
Much of the book is scientific.
Now and again I caught the meaning, which means, now and again
I was really pleased with myself as I continued to learn
about my beautiful brain.

Messengers To The Brain
"Our Fantastic Five Senses"
Paul D. Martin
National Geographic Society
This book even comes with a Classroom Activities Folder.

Neural Path Therapy
Matthew McKay, Ph.D. & David Harp, MA
"How To Change Your Brain's Response
To Anger, Fear, Pain and Desire"
A good think and the steps to get there.

The Healing Mind
Dr. Irving Oyle
"A physician looks at the mysterious ability
of the mind to heal the body"
A good look at teamwork between doctor and patient
and patient as healer.

100 Questions & Answers About Epilepsy
Anuradha Singh, MD
Thank You, Thank You, Thank You for helping me to understand
a little bit more of who I am and accept it within me.

Healing Nectar For Your Soul
40 Day Healing Guide For Your Soul
Shaheerah Stephens
The wonder of Shaheerah's book is the comforting wisdom it brings
within your soul as she guides you into the mysterious simplicity
of being the partner you are looking for through your healing journey.

Brain * The Complete Mind
Michael S. Sweeney
National Geographic
"How It Develops, How It Works, And How To Keep It Sharp"
While this book is technical
it shares the information in everyday language.
The illustrations and charts are highly beneficial.

Maps Of The Mind
Charles Hampden-Turner
"Charts and concepts of the mind and its labyrinths"
Way too technical for me yet the graphics told the story
as I needed to know it.

Saving Your Brain
Jeff Victoroff, M.D.
"The Revolutionary Plan To Boost Brain Power, Improve Memory,
and Protect Yourself Against Aging and Alzheimer's"
No pictures! Tough read yet informative.

Unicorns Are Real
Barbara Meister Vitale
"A Right-Brained Approach to Learning"
Such an interesting read for this right-brained human
who could not read until months after my first brain surgery.

Brain Videos / DVD's I Really Love

50 First Dates

Adam Sandler & Drew Barrymore

Awakenings

Robin Williams & Robert De Niro

Forrest Gump

Tom Hanks

God and Your Brain

Timothy R. Jennings, MD. FAPA

Phenomenon

John Travolta

Welcome To Marwen

Steve Carell

Brain Audio-Books I Really Like

God and the Brain

Andrew Newburg, M.D.

Meditations to Change Your Brain

Rick Hanson, Ph.D. & Richard Mendius, M.D.

Stress-Proof Your Brain

Rick Hanson, Ph.D.

The Neurobiology of WE

Daniel J. Siegel, M.D.

PART THREE

Accessories to The Book

Today I Count My "I AM" Blessings Card Deck

Start Each Card with The Intention
"Today I Count My Blessings"
Complete each card with "I AM"
The I AM Blessings Card Deck
Allows one to pick a card of their choosing by day,
several times a day and/or as unexpected emotions,
physical challenges, mental frustrations, spiritual subtleties arise.
Each card is a moment of encouragement
allowing one to re-center themselves
moving into a more
optimistic productive life affirming thought process.
Sold as a set with the book or separately at curlygirlpublications.com

Gray Wrist Band
"What My Brain Has Taught Me * Gray Matters"

Both are sold separately or as a three-part set along with the Book at
curlygirlpublications.com

Look What I Can Do!

The Start of Your Personal Journal

These twelve blank pages are but only the beginning of the unwritten of each person's life as we have never and never shall pass this way again. Practically it documents progress through healing. Through real life documentation comes self-inspiration as recording one's own struggles as well as triumphs allows reflection gauging accomplishments of yesterday, last week, a month ago, in times when it seems we have come to a standstill long enough causing discouragement, sadness, and frustration. Reading in one's own handwriting and/or scribble, no matter how shaky and as time goes on less so, about how I could not do and now a week later I can, brings a fullness expanding the heart, the mind, and the spirit to get up and do it again. Get yourself a full blank journal.

Always write your life story.

Look What I Can Do!

Look What I Can Do!

Look What I Can Do!

Look What I Can Do!

Look What I Can Do!

Look What I Can Do!

Look What I Can Do!

Look What I Can Do!

Look What I Can Do!

Look What I Can Do!

Look What I Can Do!

Look What I Can Do!

Place Your Pictures Here

Your Pictures Here frames are set into the Journal accommodating space for photographs. I told Kenny prior to my first brain surgery "No photographs. I do not want to see it." I am ever so glad he did not listen. The first time I looked at my bald, stitched head, I cried and nearly passed out yet there was a spirit of warrior, gladiator, heroine that embodied me when I saw the photos realizing that was me.

Thoughts like

I am a survivor, how is it people can survive this knowing half their head was on another table from their body, we are strong beyond our mortal knowing, came through me giving me expansive strength for that which I knew not ahead of me. He took lots of photos through my Gamma Knife Procedure so that I could share this power, this force, this courage with anyone who needed to see who they are.

Place Your Pictures Here

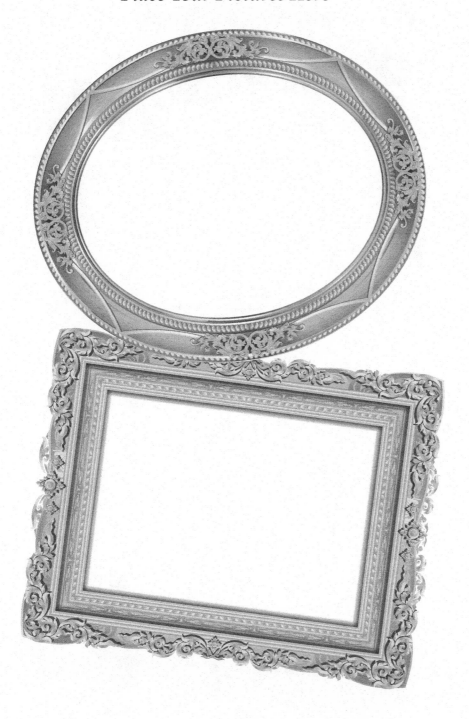

Place Your Pictures Here

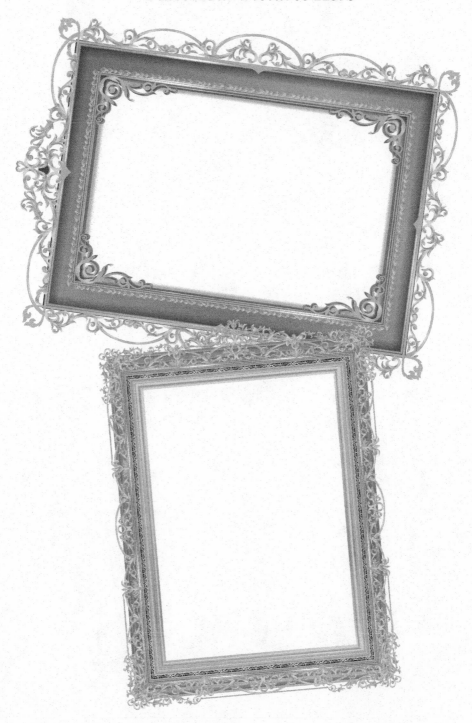

Place Your Pictures Here

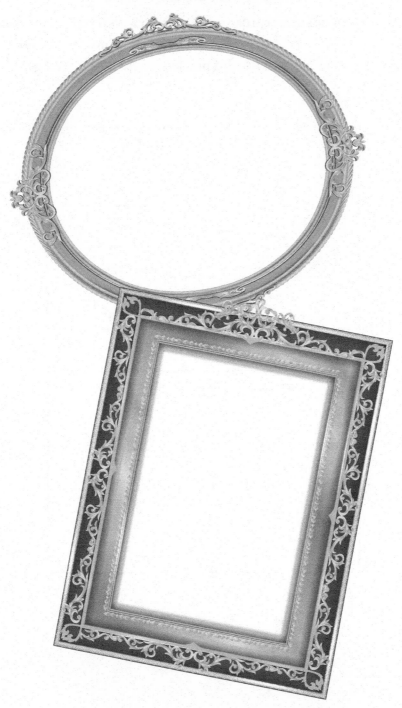

Emergency Alert Cards

Copy and cut out these cards and keep them with you in many places at all times. Give them to personal caretakers, family members and close friends to have on hand if needed.

EMERGENCY ALERT

I HAVE A BRAIN TUMOR

My Name Is _____

Tumor Type _____

I have had these treatments:

_____ Surgery _____ Chemotherapy

_____ Radiation _____ Biologic Therapy

EMERGENCY ALERT

I HAVE A BRAIN TUMOR

Emergency Contact _____

Phone Number _____

I am in a clinical trial _____ Yes _____ No

Contact This Doctor _____

Phone Number _____

EMERGENCY ALERT

I HAVE A BRAIN TUMOR

My Name Is _____

Tumor Type _____

I have had these treatments:

_____ Surgery _____ Chemotherapy

_____ Radiation _____ Biologic Therapy

EMERGENCY ALERT

I HAVE A BRAIN TUMOR

My Name Is _____

Tumor Type _____

I have had these treatments:

_____ Surgery _____ Chemotherapy

_____ Radiation _____ Biologic Therapy

EMERGENCY ALERT

I HAVE A BRAIN TUMOR

Emergency Contact _____

Phone Number _____

I am in a clinical trial _____Yes _____No

Contact This Doctor _____
    Phone Number _____

EMERGENCY ALERT

I HAVE A BRAIN TUMOR

Emergency Contact _____

Phone Number _____

I am in a clinical trial _____Yes _____No

Contact This Doctor _____
    Phone Number _____